Vitamin D

The

Sunshine

Vitamin

Vitamin D

The Sunshine Vitamin

ZOLTAN RONA, MD, MSC

The information in this book is presented for educational purposes only. It is not intended to be a substitute for the medical advice of your healthcare professional.

Published by Books Alive, an imprint of
Book Publishing Company
PO Box 99
Summertown, TN 38483
(888) 260-8458 www.bookpubco.com

Printed in Canada

15 14 13 12 11 10 9 8 7 6 5 4 3 2 1

ISBN: 978-0-920470-82-4

Library of Congress Cataloging-in-Publication Data

Rona, Zoltan P., 1951-
Vitamin D : the sunshine vitamin / Zoltan Rona.
p. cm.
ISBN 978-0-920470-82-4
1. Vitamin D. 2. Vitamin D in human nutrition. 3. Dietary supplements.
I. Title.
QP772.V53R66 2009
612.3'99--dc22

2009039841

Book Publishing Co. is a member of Green Press Initiative. We chose to print this title on paper with postconsumer recycled content and processed chlorine free, which saved the following natural resources:

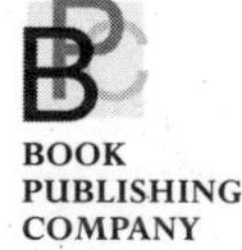

- 26 trees
- 716 pounds of solid waste
- 11,788 gallons of water
- 2,448 pounds of greenhouse gases
- 8 million BTUs of net energy

green press INITIATIVE

For more information visit: www.greenpressinitiative.org. Savings calculations from the Environmental Defense Paper Calculator <www.edf.org/papercalculator>

Contents

Sun phobia, sunscreens, and spending too much time indoors have all contributed to the problem of vitamin D insufficiency.

Introduction

It is conservatively estimated by most experts that 70 percent of the population in Canada and the United States is vitamin D deficient. In my private medical practice in Toronto, I found a very similar percentage of my patients to be vitamin D deficient as well. About five years ago, when all the newspapers were filled with the latest news and research about vitamin D, I routinely started to measure the levels of vitamin D in all my patients. To my utter surprise, the majority had suboptimal levels of the vitamin, even during the summer months. I reasoned that this was because people were frightened to death about the cancer-causing dangers of too much sun exposure and the many media pronouncements about using sunscreens, coupled with scary stories of vitamin D toxicity from oral supplements.

Sun phobia—a condition imposed on the population by sun-paranoid dermatologists—sunscreens, and spending too much time indoors due to the fear of aging from sun damage have all contributed to the problem of vitamin D insufficiency. One of the worst offenders in creating vitamin D deficiency is the use of commercial sunscreens, none of which have been proved to prevent skin cancer and most of which contain carcinogenic chemicals. Studies now indicate that while sunscreens may prevent sunburns, they do virtually nothing to prevent cancer and other illnesses.

When the June 8, 2007, front page of the *Toronto Globe and Mail* proclaimed the cancer-preventing benefits of vitamin D and the Canadian Cancer Society chirped in with their modest recommendation for everyone to take 1,100 IU of vitamin D daily, the natural health community may have felt vindicated. Many scientists felt hoodwinked.

This cancer-preventive property of vitamin D was no big news to world experts and researchers who have been touting the numerous benefits of the vitamin for well over a decade. The medical profession and its various antiquated societies are, unfortunately, far behind in applying scientific data to clinical health concerns. It's a nice gesture on their part to recommend 1,100 IU of vitamin D a day to prevent cancer, but it's far from enough. Current research indicates that the figure for cancer prevention should be closer to 10,000 IU daily. This figure will probably surface as a regular recommendation only in another decade. It's just the way the snail goes for the world of conventional medical wisdom.

But change will come. We are now seeing daily evidence of vitamin D's promise as study after scientific study is published extolling its benefits for virtually every human disease. Vitamin D deficiency and insufficiency play a role in causing seventeen types of cancer (especially of the breast, colon, and prostate) as well as autoimmune diseases like birth defects, chronic pain, depression (especially seasonal affective disorder), diabetes (Type 1 and Type 2), fibromyalgia, heart disease, hypertension, multiple sclerosis, muscle wasting, muscle weakness, obesity, osteoarthritis, osteoporosis, periodontal disease, and stroke. Furthermore, vitamin D has been proved to regulate over two thousand genes in the body, and this may be why so many diseases are directly influenced by its availability.

Vitamin D

The Sunshine Vitamin

1

Vitamin D Basics

Vitamin D is not your typical vitamin. First, vitamin D (also called the sunshine vitamin) is created under the skin by ultraviolet light. We usually get vitamins from the foods we eat; however, in the case of vitamin D, there simply are not enough rich food sources for people to get adequate amounts in their diet. To get sufficient vitamin D, we need to be exposed to sunshine or use supplements.

Second, unlike other vitamins, vitamin D is turned into a hormone in the body. This biochemically active form of vitamin D is closely related structurally to two other hormones, cortisone and estrogen.

The body has a huge need for vitamin D. All cells, tissues, and organs in the human body have vitamin D receptors, basically meaning that they await the arrival of the vitamin (or hormone) to perform various vital functions.

The most basic and best-known role of vitamin D is to regulate calcium and phosphorus metabolism; that is, vitamin D tells calcium and phosphorus where to go and what to do. Working with the parathyroid glands located in the neck, vitamin D helps the gut absorb calcium and helps to balance calcium with phosphorus in the arteries, bones, kidneys, and teeth. If calcium and phosphorus intakes are adequate and vitamin D is deficient, major problems can arise in numerous tissues and organs, leading to diseases such as atherosclerosis, blood-clotting disorders, kidney stones, osteoporosis, and at least thirty-six other diseases.

When vitamin D levels in the blood are low, both calcium and phosphorus levels decrease, causing parathormone to be released from the parathyroid glands. This, in turn, causes the bones to release calcium and phosphorus to maintain a steady state of these two minerals in the blood. When vitamin D levels in the blood are sufficient, the hormone calcitonin causes excess calcium and phosphorus to be returned to the bones. Vitamin D works to orchestrate this complex phenomenon, and sufficient levels are crucial for bone health.

Without adequate amounts of vitamin D, bones lose minerals and even mass. Low levels of calcium also affect the nervous system and the cardiovascular system. In addition, it is now known that vitamin D controls several adrenal gland hormones, the speed at which cells grow, the production of enzymes, and the function of some of our genes.

VITAMIN D IN THE HUMAN BODY

Without sunshine or a source of ultraviolet light—or in people with very dark skin—vitamin D production is significantly impaired. Vitamin D_3 (cholecalciferol) is actually manufactured in the skin when ultraviolet light, either from the sun or a tanning bed, interacts with the enzyme 7-dehydrocholesterol to form it. Then the liver and kidneys take over, converting vitamin D_3 into the major circulating, active forms of vitamin D called 25-hydroxy cholecalciferol and 1,25-dihydroxy cholecalciferol.

If vitamin D is ingested from either an animal or plant source (it exists in only minute amounts in the plant kingdom), it is absorbed through the walls of the small intestine with the aid of bile coming from the gallbladder (or the liver, in those people without gallbladders). Some conditions such as food allergies can bind vitamin D and prevent its absorption from the gut.

VITAMIN D FROM HEAD TO TOE

Vitamin D is needed for optimal health, including the following:

- adrenal gland health
- aging prevention and longevity
- blood sugar control
- bone metabolism
- brain and nervous system development and function
- digestion and nutrient absorption
- fertility
- hair follicle health
- hearing
- heart and circulation health
- immune system health
- mood, mind, memory, and behavior
- muscle, nerve, and athletic performance
- normal blood pressure
- pancreatic health
- respiratory health
- skin health
- sleeping
- vision
- weight control, especially carbohydrate and fat metabolism

Once absorbed into the bloodstream, vitamin D is taken to the liver, where it is either used up or stored. Vitamin D is also stored in the bones, brain, skin, and spleen.

FOOD SOURCES OF VITAMIN D

Although people with vitamin D deficiency are often told to drink two glasses of milk each day during the winter months, one study published in June 2002 by the *American Journal of Medicine* concluded that drinking milk did not raise the blood levels of vitamin D. Either the degree of fortification of milk and dairy products is inadequate or the absorption of vitamin D from milk is poor for most people.

The vitamin D used to fortify milk is vitamin D_2 (ergocalciferol). This is a synthetic form of vitamin D that is also used to fortify almond milk, hemp milk, soymilk, other plant milks, margarine, and orange juice. In nature, vitamin D_2 sources are found only in plants and are very rare, but both mushrooms and dark green leafy vegetables do contain some. Vitamin D_2 can also be obtained by eating various algae (such as blue-green algae, chlorella, and spirulina), although the levels of D are very low in these too.

The other form of vitamin D is D_3 (cholecalciferol), which is the kind your body produces as the result of sun exposure; it is also found in some foods. Food sources of vitamin D_3 are all nonvegan and include butter, egg yolks, and oily fish like herring, mackerel, salmon, and sardines.

Throughout this book, I refer to both forms simply as vitamin D unless it is important to specify one form or the other.

TABLE 1: SOME FOOD SOURCES OF VITAMIN D

Food	IUs per serving*	Percent DV**
Cod liver oil, 1 tablespoon	1,360	340
Salmon, cooked, 3.5 ounces	360	90
Mackerel, cooked, 3.5 ounces	345	90
Tuna fish, canned in oil, 3 ounces	200	50
Sardines, canned in oil, drained, 1.75 ounces	250	70
Vitamin D–fortified plant milks (made from almonds, hazelnuts, hempseeds, oats, or soy), 1 cup	100-160	25-45
Vitamin D-fortified cow's milk (nonfat, reduced fat, and whole), 1 cup	98	25
Vitamin D-fortified margarine, 1 tablespoon	60	15
Ready-to-eat cereal, fortified with vitamin D (more heavily fortified cereals might provide more of the DV), 0.75-1 cup	40	10
Egg (vitamin D is found in yolk), 1	20	6
Beef liver, cooked 3.5 ounces	15	4
Cheese, Swiss, 1 ounce	12	4

Sources: National Institutes of Health, http://ods.od.nih.gov/factsheets/vitamind.asp and *The Vegetarian Journal*, April 1, 2009, by Reed Mangels, www.accessmylibrary.com/coms2/summary_0286-37644546_ITM.

*IUs = International Units.

**DV = Daily Value. DVs were developed by the U.S. Food and Drug Administration to help consumers compare the nutrient contents of products within the context of a total diet. The DV for vitamin D is 400 IU for adults and children ages four and older. Food labels, however, are not required to list vitamin D content unless a food has been fortified with this nutrient. Foods providing 20% or more of the DV are considered to be high sources of a nutrient.

ARE YOU AT RISK?

Certain people are at greater risk for developing vitamin D deficiency:

- People who are overweight have a relatively greater need because vitamin D is stored in the body's fat cells. Therefore, a person who has more fat cells needs more vitamin D to maintain vitamin D storage levels in the body. This need is dictated by the percentage of body fat rather than body weight. Simply put, the greater your amount of body fat, the higher your vitamin D level has to be.
- Pregnant women have a greater need because they are acquiring greater body mass during pregnancy and the fetus has high nutrient demands.
- Older people can easily become vitamin D deficient because skin loses the ability to create vitamin D as it ages. It can also be argued that older people spend less time outdoors and that the quality of our nutritional intake declines as we age.
- Dark-skinned people, who have a high skin content of melanin, a pigment that blocks ultraviolet B (UVB) rays, are much more prone to vitamin D deficiency. In my private medical practice, nearly 100 percent of my African Canadian patients have low blood levels of vitamin D.

All cells, tissues, and organs in the human body have vitamin D receptors, meaning that they await the arrival of the vitamin to perform various vital functions.

2

Can you imagine what would happen if a drug company came out with a single pill that reduces the risk of cancer, heart attack, stroke, osteoporosis, PMS, SAD, and various autoimmune disorders? There would be a media frenzy the likes of which has never been seen before! Well, guess what? Such a drug exists . . . it is the sun.

—Michael Holick, physician, researcher, author, and vitamin D expert

Sunshine Is the Best Source

The best and most natural way to ensure that you are getting an adequate amount of vitamin D is to expose your skin to the sun regularly. In the northern United States, all of Canada, and other areas in northern latitudes (those above 40 degrees north), this is next to impossible at any time other than the summer. As discussed earlier, drinking milk is not the answer. Although frowned upon by overly cautious dermatologists, I recommend people use a sunbed (avoiding sunburn) during the winter months. Either that or make frequent trips to Florida, southern California, or the Caribbean.

If you live in climates where significant amounts of sunshine are unavailable for many months at a time (such as Canada and the northern United States) and you are unable to move to Hawaii, one alternative is to use tanning beds that supply ultraviolet B (UVB) rays. This is the type of ray you need to manufacture your own vitamin D. Since your body has a built-in regulation system for manufacturing just the right amounts of vitamin D, this is the optimal way that you can get it into your bloodstream.

Sitting by a window or in your car with the sun shining through glass will do nothing for your vitamin D levels because the rays must directly

VITAMIN D WHERE THE SUN DON'T SHINE

External conditions such as time of day, cloud cover, and smog can affect how much vitamin D you synthesize as a result of sun exposure. Another critical factor is where you live. Because of the angle of the sun's rays, people at northern latitudes cannot get sufficient vitamin D exposure during certain months of the year. Here is what the research tells us:

- In Edmonton, Alberta, Canada, at roughly 52 degrees north, sun exposure is not sufficient for vitamin D production from October through March.
- In Boston, Massachusetts, at roughly 42 degrees north, sun exposure is not sufficient for vitamin D production from November through February.
- Farther south, near Atlanta, Georgia, at roughly 34 degrees north, sunlight exposure is sufficient for vitamin D production in the middle of winter.

touch your skin to have any effect. If you open the windows (as long as it's not too polluted outside), you will then get the rays you need. Your bare skin needs to be exposed to direct sunlight for at least fifteen minutes each day to produce enough vitamin D to meet your needs. Windows, clothing, and various lotions all block the beneficial rays, and sunscreen prevents the manufacture of vitamin D.

We need exposure to UVB rays to manufacture our own vitamin D.

THE SUNSCREEN MYTH

For years, dermatologists and other doctors have been telling patients that sun exposure causes skin cancer and have advised them to use sunscreens and wear protective glasses, hats, and other clothing. It is thought that the higher the sun protection factor (SPF) in the sunscreen, the better. But is this correct?

The truth is that the benefits of ultraviolet light have been underestimated, while its dangers have been grossly exaggerated. Evidence in the medical journals and in the news media about the benefits of exposing bare skin to ultraviolet light is reported practically every day. For example, on February 5, 2005, the BBC News reported that more sunshine helps melanoma patients because their tumors become less aggressive. Non-Hodgkin's lymphoma is another type of cancer that can be helped by increased exposure to ultraviolet rays. In this case, the risks of developing the disease are reduced by up to 40 percent with exposure to either the sun or ultraviolet-producing sunlamps. The studies concluded that cancer rates decreased because the skin produced much more vitamin D from the increased ultraviolet light exposure.

The benefits of ultraviolet light have been underestimated, while its dangers have been grossly exaggerated.

It is important to realize that it is ultraviolet A (UVA) light and not UVB light that is responsible for skin damage, aging, and wrinkles. UVA rays are also thought to cause cancer, while UVB rays create vitamin D, which protects the body from melanoma and other skin cancers. Additional differences between UVA and UVB are highlighted in a study published by Dianne Godar of the U.S. Food and Drug Administration. For example, UVA light is able to pass through window glass, making you vulnerable even when indoors. UVB light cannot travel through glass. UVB light is strongest between 10:00 a.m. and 2:00 p.m., whereas UVA is stronger at other times. To maximize vitamin D production, most people need ten to twenty minutes of sun exposure between 10:00 a.m. and 2:00 p.m. Beyond that, unless your skin color is fairly dark, you risk some sun damage and even burns. Both UVA and UVB can cause sunburn.

It is important to realize that it is UVA light and not UVB light that is responsible for skin damage, aging, and wrinkles.

Sunlight in the early morning or latter part of the day (before 10:00 a.m. or after 2:00 p.m.) is mostly UVA. Therefore, exposure at these times is actually more dangerous in terms of cancer risk. If you are exposed to the sun when UVA rays are predominant, you are more likely to get any type of skin cancer than you would be if you limit sun exposure to the hours between 10:00 a.m. and 2:00 p.m., when UVB rays are prominent.

Most people need ten to twenty minutes of sun exposure between 10:00 a.m. and 2:00 p.m.

SUNSCREENS, SUN EXPOSURE, AND CANCER RISK

Despite all the very positive studies on the benefits of UVB, we are a society that is frightened of sunshine. We slather on chemical sunscreens in the belief that we will ward off skin cancer, even though no proof exists. Dermatologists praise the use of these sunscreens, telling the public to use products with the highest possible SPF. Moreover, they encourage us to avoid the sun, tanning beds, and vitamin supplements of any kind because, as they say, "You can get all your vitamins from your diet." All this is based on outdated information. There is no plausible evidence that the most dangerous form of skin cancer, melanoma, has anything to do with sun damage. Basal cell carcinoma (BCC), the most common form of skin cancer, is extremely benign and rarely, if ever, spreads. It is usually seen in fair-skinned people and is causally related to excess sun exposure in susceptible individuals.

There is no plausible evidence that the most dangerous form of skin cancer, melanoma, has anything to do with sun damage.

The same can be said for a less common form of skin cancer, squamous cell carcinoma. Various sunscreens might protect you against BCC and squamous cell cancer of the skin, but not melanoma. Recent studies indicate that one cause of melanoma is vitamin D deficiency and a low omega-3 to omega-6 fatty acid ratio. You can rebalance your omega fatty acid ratio by getting more ultraviolet light exposure or using supplements of omega-3 fatty acid. One recent study showed a 40 percent reduction in melanoma in frequent fish eaters. If the mercury content of fish worries you, know that most fish-oil supplements are free of mercury. If you prefer a vegetarian option, use flaxseed oil, hempseed oil, or DHA supplements from algae.

Since 1940, the incidence of melanoma has increased, mostly occurring in people who work indoors. Outdoor workers rarely get the disease and, on average, get nine times more solar radiation than their indoor counterparts. Outdoor workers make more vitamin D, which protects them from all sorts of cancers, including melanoma, provided they avoid commercial sunscreens. While the sun does cause skin damage, our bodies have developed a way of repairing this damage by creating more vitamin D under the skin. Vitamin D repairs the DNA in genes and prevents cells from mutating into cancer. Avoiding sunshine or using sunscreens negates this built-in cancer protection. Interestingly, melanoma also tends to occur in areas of the body that are less exposed to the sun or are usually covered by clothing.

Although there are some studies that show a causal relationship between sunbed tanning and increased risk of malignant melanoma, one of the largest studies on the subject, done in 2005, indicated that sunbed use has a small protective effect against melanoma. The strongest risk factors for developing melanoma are skin type (the paler the skin, the greater risk) and the number of moles present on the body. Sunscreens have no preventive value against malignant melanoma.

Oddly enough, some studies indicate that using sunscreen increases the risk of developing melanoma. In a 2007 study, subjects using sunscreen had three times the risk compared to those who never used sunscreen. People who took thirty sunbaths per year were ten times less likely to have melanoma compared with those who took less than twenty sunbaths per year. There was no such protective effect if sunburns occurred.

If you have melanoma, should you risk sunbathing or avoid the sun? While staying out of the sun might prevent premature aging and relatively benign or rare forms of skin cancer, one recent study indicates that safe levels of sun exposure can lower a melanoma patient's risk of dying. A safe approach is to limit sun exposure to fifteen minutes a day between the hours of 10:00 a.m. and 2:00 p.m. and balance blood levels with supplements as needed. Vitamin D levels plummet with less sun exposure, so cancer has a better chance of taking hold; higher blood levels of vitamin D make melanoma less aggressive. However, there is no evidence that melanoma survival rates are improved significantly with greater exposure to sunlight. If your doctor or anyone else tells you to stay out of the sun, mention these facts and ask for evidence to the contrary.

For people who must spend hours in the sun due to the nature of their work, the safest sunscreen to use to prevent damage or sunburn is one that blocks both UVA and UVB rays. However, most sunscreens block the potentially beneficial UVB rays, which help produce vitamin D, while allowing the more damaging UVA rays to come through, and it is UVA light that appears to be associated with a greater risk of melanoma. The majority of recently published scientific papers indicate that a greater risk exists for melanoma with decreased sun exposure and subsequent low blood levels of vitamin D. The end result is that use of commercial sunscreens with any SPF factor can produce a higher cancer risk due to vitamin D deficiency.

Since 1940, the incidence of melanoma has increased, mostly occurring in people who work indoors.

SMART CHOICES IN THE SUN

Pursuing the health benefits of sun exposure does not mean that you should stay out long enough to get sunburned. Suntanning does not mean sunburning. Never allow yourself to burn. If you have not been exposed to sunlight in months, go out for ten minutes a day until your skin becomes accustomed to the ultraviolet rays. When you see your skin turning a bit pink, it's time to head for the shade. Over time, skin gradually turns darker with more sun exposure. As your skin tans, you will be able to spend more time in the sun because darker skin tones offer more ultraviolet light protection.

In summary, to avoid sunburn use natural sunscreens that contain either titanium dioxide or zinc oxide. For burns, use aloe vera lotion or zinc oxide cream. My recommendation is to avoid commercial sunscreens, which are more likely to contain carcinogenic chemicals. Recent research has shown that many of these sunscreens are not effective and may even be harmful. For example, 2009 research by the Environmental Working Group showed that of 1,606 sunscreens tested, three out of five offered inadequate sun protection or actually contained toxic ingredients. If you want to avoid sunscreens, you can use clothing, floppy hats, sunglasses, and an umbrella, since these are all more likely to be effective at preventing sunburn.

Suntanning does not mean sunburning. Never allow yourself to burn.

CHECK SUNSCREEN INGREDIENTS CAREFULLY

Aside from the vitamin D deficiency created by sunscreen use, many of the chemicals commonly found in these products are potentially carcinogenic. About 90 percent contain octyl methoxycinnamate, which can turn extremely toxic when exposed to sunlight. It's safe to say that if you cannot pronounce it or eat it, you probably shouldn't put it on your skin. **Here are the sunscreen ingredients to avoid:**

- avobenzone
- dioxybenzone
- homosalate
- methyl anthranilate
- octocrylene
- octyl methoxycinnamate
- oxybenzone (2-hydroxy-4-methoxybenzophenone)
- PABA (para-aminobenzoic acid)
- padimate A
- padimate O
- phenylbenzimidazole
- sulisobenzone
- trolamine salicylate
- 2-ethylhexyl p-methoxycinnamate
- 2-ethylhexyl salicylate, octyl salicylate, and other forms of salicylic acid (aspirin)

By the way, dioxybenzone and oxybenzone are two of the most powerful free radical generators ever formulated in a laboratory. Check labels very carefully.

The best natural ingredients that block both UVA and UVB rays are titanium dioxide and zinc oxide. Other ingredients that are often used in "natural" commercial sunscreens and that are safe to use include the following:

- aloe vera
- coconut oil
- eucalyptus oil
- glycerin
- jojoba oil
- lecithin
- shea butter
- sunflower seed oil
- vitamin E (tocopherol)

Unfortunately, even these natural sunscreens prevent skin from manufacturing adequate levels of vitamin D.

VITAMIN D DOWN THE DRAIN

One last point must be made for anyone concerned about getting enough vitamin D from exposure to sunshine. We know that vitamin D is formed when skin is exposed to UVB radiation from the sun or a tanning bed. The vitamin D formed in this way does not immediately travel through the skin into the bloodstream. This process takes up to forty-eight hours. Showering and scrubbing your skin within forty-eight hours of exposure could conceivably wash away the vitamin D on the skin's surface and prevent absorption into the bloodstream. This may be why so many people are vitamin D deficient despite hours of sun exposure. They may actually be wiping away the vitamin D long before it can be absorbed.

Showering only every two days is not realistic, particularly if you live in a warmer climate. You can still shower daily, rinsing the entire body with warm water and using soap principally on the underarms, genitals, and feet; just take care not to scrub off the vitamin D from your arms and legs.

Showering and scrubbing your skin within forty-eight hours of exposure could conceivably wash away the vitamin D on the skin's surface and prevent absorption into the bloodstream.

3

Vitamin D Supplements

If you want nothing to do with sunbeds or trips to the tropics, vitamin D supplements will do the trick. Both vitamin D_2 and D_3 supplements are available.

There is considerable controversy among vitamin D experts about the safety and effectiveness of oral supplementation with vitamin D_2 (ergocalciferol) versus vitamin D_3 (cholecalciferol). The basic difference between the two forms has to do with how they are manufactured. Vitamin D_2 is derived from vegetarian sources, manufactured through the action of ultraviolet light on ergosterol from yeast. Vitamin D_3, on the other hand, is manufactured from a cholesterol derivative from lanolin (an animal source). Vitamin D_2 is cheaper and easier to make and has been used to fortify foods and make supplements.

Some of the world's leading experts, like Rheinhold Vieth, associate professor at the University of Toronto, believe that vitamin D_2 is less effective than D_3. In a paper titled "The Case Against Ergocalciferol (Vitamin D_2) as a Vitamin Supplement," published in 2006 in the *American Journal of Clinical Nutrition*, Vieth and coauthor Lisa Houghton conclude that vitamin D_2 should not be considered the equivalent of vitamin D_3. They claim that vitamin D_2 behaves differently in the body, creates different metabolic by-products, and may be more difficult for the body to eliminate. They also claim that the shelf life of vitamin D_2 is shorter than that of vitamin D_3 and that this diminishes its potency and effectiveness.

According to the Vitamin D Council, vitamin D_2 is two to four times less effective than D_3 and produces potentially toxic metabolites. The following comes from the vitamin D Council website: "[Vitamin] D_2 (ergocalciferol) is not human vitamin D, it may be a weaker agonist, it is not normally present in humans, and its consumption results in metabolic by-products not normally found in humans. It is also two to four times less effective than D_3 (cholecalciferol) in raising 25(OH)D levels."

Michael Holick, another leading medical researcher and expert on vitamin D, has concluded the opposite based on different data. His research at Boston University was published in 2008 and determined that the actions of vitamin D_2 were the same as those of vitamin D_3. According to Holick, "1,000 IU of vitamin D_2 daily was as effective as 1,000 IU of vitamin D_3 in maintaining serum 25-hydroxy vitamin D levels [the active

TEST YOUR VITAMIN D BLOOD LEVELS

As you will be consistently reminded as you read this book, I highly recommend blood tests for vitamin D levels. I order regular blood tests for my patients who are using vitamin D supplements. Here is the information you need to know about testing for vitamin D levels:

- Ask your doctor to check your blood level of 25-hydroxy vitamin D, sometimes referred to as 25(OH)D. Do not use the 1,25-dihydroxy test, which is not as accurate. In addition, check ionized calcium levels.
- Get tested every three months.
- Optimal 25-hydroxy vitamin D blood levels should be between 100 and 250 ng/ml. Levels below 50 are considered insufficient. Levels below 25 are definitely in the deficiency category.
- As research on vitamin D continues, I predict these numbers will all change, so stay tuned.

form found in the bloodstream] and did not negatively influence serum 25-hydroxy vitamin D levels. Therefore, vitamin D_2 is equally as effective as vitamin D_3 in maintaining 25-hydroxy vitamin D status." In other words, vitamin D_2 supplements work every bit as well in maintaining adequate blood levels of vitamin D.

It's difficult to make a definitive conclusion about the use of vitamin D_2, especially when such contrasting expert opinions exist. At present, unless I am proven wrong by new research on the subject, my conclusion is that vitamin D_2 is as safe and effective as D_3 as a supplement. Blood testing will certainly tell you whether or not you are getting adequate blood levels, regardless of the type and amount of vitamin D supplement you are using.

My conclusion is that vitamin D_2 is as safe and effective as vitamin D_3 as a supplement.

DOSING AND TOXICITY FEARS

One of the universal truths (or myths) we were all taught in medical school thirty or more years ago was that fat-soluble vitamins like vitamin D were toxic at certain levels. It was said that daily doses of over 2,000 IU would elevate blood levels of calcium, damage the kidneys irreversibly, and lead to generalized atherosclerosis (hardening of the arteries). To this day, I still hear conventional medical doctors regurgitating these same fears to their patients.

Scientists from around the world are now coming to the conclusion that the old recommended daily allowance (RDA) for vitamin D of 400 IU is no longer the valid minimum requirement and is insufficient except for achieving the minimal goal of preventing rickets. In June 2007, in a flurry of generosity, even the highly conservative Canadian Cancer Society recommended that we all supplement with 1,100 IU daily of vitamin D. Unfortunately, a daily dose of 1,000 IU will do nothing to correct a deficiency. According to Reinhold Vieth, researcher at the University of Toronto, blood levels don't even measurably rise until 4,000 IU (100 micrograms) is consumed. Real toxicity (hypercalcemia and rampant atherosclerosis) begins at 40,000 IU (1,000 micrograms, or 1 milligram) only after many weeks of use.

Research now indicates that the correct figure for the minimum daily requirement is 4,000 IU. It will probably take another decade before the government nutritional authorities acknowledge this fact and recommend much higher vitamin D intakes for the population.

Research also indicates that to get 4,000 IU of vitamin D daily if you totally avoid the sun, you must drink forty glasses of fortified milk a day or take ten typical multivitamin pills daily. I consider 10,000 IU to be the optimal daily dose of vitamin D. At that dose, I have never seen anyone run into side effects or toxicity symptoms in over thirty years.

My advice, and it's quite conservative, is for all Canadians and Americans living in northern latitudes (above 40 degrees north) to supplement with a bare minimum of 4,000 IU of vitamin D daily during the winter months. This is especially true for pregnant women who have a family history of multiple sclerosis or cancer, just to name a couple of diseases that can be prevented by vitamin D supplements.

Most individuals will see some benefit with vitamin D supplements within three or four months but, since there is a great genetic variation in terms of vitamin D metabolism from person to person, the changes may be evident either earlier or much later. The best way to monitor the safety and effectiveness of supplements, as well as how much you may need at any given time, is with periodic blood tests.

In the summer, provided you get adequate sunshine (at least ten to twenty minutes a day), you may not need supplements and no monitoring is really necessary because the body monitors and adjusts blood levels of vitamin D automatically. For example, if you are out in the sun for over five hours, you could theoretically be making 100,000 units of vitamin D under your exposed skin. Despite this, blood levels will adjust so that vitamin D levels remain stable. If you then stay out of the sun for many days, skin reserves of vitamin D will be moved into your bloodstream slowly to normalize levels there. This sort of thing will not happen with oral supplements and, if you supplement with doses much higher than 4,000 IU daily, the potential for toxicity is there. So, as a general rule, if you supplement at very high doses for any length of time, get blood testing for 25-hydroxy vitamin D done at least every three months.

I consider 10,000 IU to be the optimal daily dose of vitamin D. At that dose, I have never seen anyone run into side effects or toxicity symptoms in over thirty years.

HARVARD MEDICAL SCHOOL RECOMMENDS VITAMIN D SUPPLEMENTS

Here is a surprising but welcome statement made by a conservative group of academics that usually recommends that people get their vitamins from the food they eat rather than supplements. The September 2009 issue of the *Harvard Health Publications Bulletin* of Harvard Medical School stated that taking vitamin D supplements was the key to achieving vitamin D adequacy. The statement said: "Even a low-calorie diet can deliver all the vitamins and minerals you need, with one exception—vitamin D. So plan to take a vitamin D supplement. You can't get much from foods. You can get it through sunlight, but it's a lot easier to go ahead and take a supplement. . . . While some experts may think it ideal that we get all the nutrients we need from food alone, the fact of the matter is that the majority of Americans don't always eat as well as they should."

SHOULD YOU MEGADOSE WITH VITAMIN D?

Some of you might be surprised to know that there are many physicians in both Canada and the United States who prescribe as much as 50,000 IU of vitamin D daily as a treatment for a long list of chronic diseases. According to the world research authorities on vitamin D, the Vitamin D Council, fears of high-dose vitamin D are irrational. To quote the Vitamin D Council from their website: "The single most important fact anyone needs to know about vitamin D is how much nature supplies if we behave naturally, e.g., go into the sun. Humans make at least 10,000 units of vitamin D within thirty minutes of full-body exposure to the sun, what is called a minimal erythemal dose. Vitamin D production in the skin occurs within minutes and is already maximized before your skin turns pink."

Reinhold Vieth says, "Fear of vitamin D toxicity is unwarranted, and such unwarranted fear, bordering on hysteria, is rampant in the medical profession. If there is published evidence of toxicity in adults from an intake of 250 μg (10,000 IU) per day, and that is verified by the 25(OH)D concentration, I have yet to find it."

Physician and author Jonathan Wright of the Tahoma Clinic in Washington State says, "It's very likely that if you're over forty and supplement your diet with a generous amount of vitamin D, you can lower your risk of prostate, breast, and bowel cancer, along with your risk of 'essential' hypertension, osteoporosis, and tuberculosis."

I first learned about high-dose vitamin D therapy from one of Norm Shealy's newsletters (www.normshealy.com). Norm Shealy is a physician, the author of several books, and the founder of the American Holistic Medical Association. Shealy relates, "Recently I had the good fortune to spend a couple of hours with Joe Prendergast, an endocrinologist and diabetologist. He has managed over fifteen hundred diabetic patients and, in the last decade, not one of his patients has had a stroke or heart attack. Only one has even been hospitalized! His secret—50,000 units of vitamin D_3 daily."

Joe Prendergast, a California physician and author, further reports these benefits from large doses of vitamin D:

- control of many cancers, including breast cancer, brain tumors, colon cancer, leukemia, myeloma, and prostate cancer
- cure of amyotrophic lateral sclerosis (ALS)
- cure of depression and many other mental disorders
- cure of Hashimoto's thyroiditis
- cure of multiple sclerosis (MS)
- improvement in allergies
- prevention of influenza
- regression of rheumatoid arthritis
- reversal of advanced coronary disease
- reversal of advanced lung disease, avoiding lung transplant
- reversal of osteoporosis

Shealy also has this to say: "Most of you know that I personally take 50,000 units of D_3 daily and have for eighteen months. I recommend it to most people who weigh at least 140 pounds or more and take no calcium supplements. One of my audience informed me that he developed a very high blood calcium that affected his kidneys. I have not been able to learn whether he took calcium supplements. But, if you do the daily D_3, I would advise a blood calcium level at three months and at six-month intervals. I have not seen this in hundreds of others, but be advised."

John Cannell, physician and head of the Vitamin D Council, recommends doses as high as 50,000 IU daily for quickly getting rid of a cold or flu but has not generally advocated such high doses. One of the problems with supplementing with such high doses of vitamin D is the effect it may have on calcium, specifically the deposit of calcium in the arteries and organs. Apparently, this is a problem only if you are also taking high calcium doses as a supplement. In any event, if you decide to supplement with high doses of vitamin D, make sure that blood tests are done every three months to check calcium levels.

Fear of vitamin D toxicity is unwarranted, and such unwarranted fear, bordering on hysteria, is rampant in the medical profession.

Treating Vitamin D Toxicity

In the 1930s and 1940s, doctors prescribed up to 600,000 IU of vitamin D to treat arthritis. Following one 1948 study, Johns Hopkins University reported that ten patients developed vitamin D toxicity after taking massive doses of vitamin D. The amounts used in the study ranged from 150,000 to 600,000 IU daily, and toxic symptoms occurred after two to eighteen months.

The side effects of taking these huge doses of vitamin D included weight loss and fatigue, followed by anorexia, nausea, and vomiting. All subjects had high blood calcium levels and kidney damage. Nine out of ten were anemic, but seven out of ten claimed that their arthritis was much better on the high doses. Those who reported an improvement in arthritis symptoms saw a return of joint pain several months after discontinuing the vitamin D supplementation. These complaints coincided closely with the return to normal blood calcium levels.

The 1948 study reported no deaths. Deaths from vitamin D toxicity have been reported in the literature, but these deaths occurred only when doctors used high-dose corticosteroids as a treatment to speed recovery from vitamin D toxicity.

The treatments needed to reverse toxicity are simple: stop taking vitamin D supplements, stay out of the sun, and drink at least four liters of water a day. The clinical symptoms of vitamin D toxicity disappear in several weeks. The blood calcium level becomes normal again after several months. The kidney damage also reverses but takes several more months.

The treatments needed to reverse vitamin D toxicity are simple: stop taking vitamin D supplements, stay out of the sun, and drink at least four liters of water a day.

PRECAUTIONS

Some legitimate precautions must be taken to prevent the rare possibility that vitamin D supplements can cause damage. Elevated calcium levels can cause atherosclerosis (hardening of the arteries), calcium deposits in the joints, and kidney stones. Here are some situations that require extra attention and, of course, routine blood testing of vitamin D blood levels:

• Many adults use statin drugs—such as Crestor (rosuvastatin calcium), Lipitor (atorvastatin), Pravachol (pravastatin sodium), and Zocor (simvastatin)—to lower blood levels of cholesterol. Since vitamin D is manufactured under the skin from cholesterol, low cholesterol levels created by statin drugs may actually create a vitamin D deficiency. Anyone taking cholesterol-lowering drugs of any kind should definitely keep getting their blood levels of vitamin D monitored.

• Some prescription drugs are known to deplete the body of vitamin D and lead to bone loss and numerous other diseases. Examples of such drugs are steroids like prednisone, Cortef (hydrocortisone), Decadron (dexamethasone), and dozens of others. The weight-loss drugs Alli and Xenical (orlistat) block fat absorption and may actually create a vitamin D deficiency. The cholesterol-lowering drug Questran (cholestyramine) has a similar effect. The antiepilepsy drugs Dilantin (phenytoin) and phenobarbital increase the liver metabolism of vitamin D, making for a speedier excretion of the vitamin from the body. These then lead to both vitamin D and calcium deficiencies.

• Vitamin D can theoretically interact with antacids containing aluminum and with numerous drugs. This does not mean that antacid users should not supplement with vitamin D. Rather, the vitamin should be consumed at least two hours before or after the drug has been administered, and the blood levels of both vitamin D and calcium should be monitored more regularly.

• For someone with severe kidney disease (renal failure), vitamin D levels could conceivably escalate to the point that dangerously high calcium levels are achieved.

• In cases of hyperparathyroidism (overactive parathyroid gland), calcium levels may already be elevated as a result of a tumor of the parathyroid gland. In such cases, vitamin D supplements should be used with caution but may actually cause a normalization of the blood levels of calcium.

• In cases of lymphoma, vitamin D supplements can raise calcium levels and lead to kidney stone formation. Use vitamin D cautiously.

• Vitamin D at virtually any supplement level can abnormally elevate blood calcium levels in those suffering from sarcoidosis. The same is true for a rare disease called histoplasmosis.

Some good news is that there are no known adverse interactions between vitamin D and foods.

Since vitamin D is manufactured under the skin from cholesterol, low cholesterol levels created by statin drugs may actually create a vitamin D deficiency.

DOCTORS STILL FEAR VITAMIN D TOXICITY

Here is a letter I recently received that illustrates the confusion that exists within the medical profession about vitamin D toxicity:

Dear Dr. Rona:
"Oh God, no" was the response when a young friend of mine told a doctor at Toronto's St. Michael's Hospital MS clinic that she was taking 14,000 IU of vitamin D a day. "There is no long-term evidence that it does not cause harm to the immune system. We don't know what blood level has to do with toxicity." She was further told to follow *Canada's Food Guide* and "eat whatever you want" when she asked about food allergies and allergy tests. (Her GP considers allergy tests unnecessary!) As you know, this sort of stuff goes against a great deal of published scientific information.

She is now afraid to take the 14,000 IU daily dose. Her mother was a pharmacist and seems to agree.

This MS clinic is apparently one of the largest in the world and, according to their web page, it's the largest clinical trial and research center in the world. I happened upon a fund-raising function for the clinic and did not pick up the promotional literature because of a prominent pharmaceutical company logo.

So there. We all now understand that vitamin D is more dangerous than pharmaceuticals in the treatment of MS. This is very strange indeed, or is it?
–Anonymous

My reply to her follows:

Dear Anonymous:
Staying out in the sun every day for two hours makes close to 20,000 IU of vitamin D. Where are all the dead bodies from that? If those uninformed practitioners had read the literature, especially anything written by Rheinhold Vieth or Michael Holick, they would talk differently and be really able to help people. Drugs are not the only way to treat MS. I'm sure your research will find numerous articles that basically say the same thing. Please tell your friend not to get scared off taking her vitamin D supplement and to get her 25-hydroxy vitamin D and ionized calcium levels checked. If the vitamin D is above 250 and below 600, with the ionized calcium in the normal range, she is on adequate doses. Otherwise, adjust the doses accordingly.
–Dr. Rona

SHOPPING FOR A SUPPLEMENT

Many vitamin D supplements, both vitamin D_2 and D_3, are readily available. These usually come in dosages of 400 IU or 1,000 IU per capsule. In Canada, higher potencies per capsule are available by prescription only.

Problems with Vitamin D from Fish Oil

If you prefer D_3 and choose cod liver oil or halibut liver oil liquid or capsules, keep in mind that a high amount of vitamin A accompanies vitamin D when these two vitamins are packaged in the same capsule. Each capsule may contain as much as 5,000 IU of vitamin A along with 200–400 IU of vitamin D. If you want to take 2,000 IU daily of vitamin D, this might be suitable. If you want to push the dose up to 10,000 IU of vitamin D daily, you might be getting too much vitamin A. For people who hate taking pills of any kind or who have problems absorbing fat-soluble vitamins (such as A, D, E, and K), supplements are available in liquid form but may be obtainable only with a prescription.

When you take oral nutritional supplements, there is no mechanism in play to keep vitamin D at safe blood levels as there is when you get your vitamin D from sunshine. If you are suffering from any chronic health problem, ask your doctor to check your blood level of 25-hydroxy vitamin D, the most accurate indicator of vitamin D status.

Rocaltrol

Rocaltrol (calcitriol) is a synthetic mimic (analogue) of vitamin D prescribed by doctors to regulate the absorption of calcium from the gastrointestinal tract. Rocaltrol is primarily used for people who have kidney failure and who are not yet on dialysis. It is also prescribed to treat an overactive parathyroid gland. Those who suffer from kidney failure cannot convert 25-hydroxy vitamin D to the active form of vitamin D_3. The capsules are either 0.25 mcg or 0.5 mcg dosages. Unfortunately, they contain butylated hydroxyanisole (BHA) and butylated hydroxytoluene (BHT) as antioxidants. The chemically sensitive individual may not tolerate this product, which also contains some potential carcinogens in the form of FD&C Red No. 3, FD&C Yellow No. 6, and other additives. The other issue with this rightfully termed "drug" is that it is considerably more expensive than any over-the-counter vitamin D supplement.

4

Diseases That Are Prevented and Treated by Vitamin D

Let's look at some of the many illnesses that would either be prevented or improved substantially in people who had optimal vitamin D blood levels. Vitamin D plays a vital role in at least two thousand genes responsible for disease prevention. It should therefore not be too surprising that it can have a huge effect on our health and even whether we live or die.

Vitamin D may as well be called the anti-death vitamin. That's because a study done in 2008 was able to show that the risk of death from all causes can be decreased by 26 percent with vitamin D supplementation. The study was published in the *Archives of Internal Medicine*, a publication of the American Medical Association.

The study followed 13,331 healthy men and women for nine years, during which time 1,806 deaths occurred. Of these deaths, nearly seven hundred were associated with heart disease, and four hundred of these subjects were deficient in vitamin D. When the 25-hydroxy vitamin D blood levels in all study participants were compared, it was found that those with the highest levels had a 26 percent lower chance of dying. The cause of death (such as cancer or heart disease) did not make any difference. The crucial factor was the blood level of vitamin D.

The researchers reported, "Our results make it much more clear that all men and women concerned about their overall health should more closely monitor their blood levels of vitamin D, and make sure they have enough."

In addition, they said, "We think we have additional evidence to consider adding vitamin D deficiency as a distinct and separate risk factor for death from cardiovascular disease, putting it alongside much better known and understood risk factors such as age, gender, family history, smoking, high blood cholesterol levels, high blood pressure, lack of exercise, obesity, and diabetes."

Because of the large role vitamin D plays not only in cardiovascular disease but also in cancer and autoimmune diseases, I devote separate sections to these topics. Following those is an alphabetical listing of the many other conditions that can be affected by vitamin D.

Vitamin D may as well be called the anti-death vitamin.

CANCER

Approximately 70 percent of Canadians and Americans are vitamin D deficient. As a direct result of this deficiency, about two million North Americans will die from cancer each year.

Vitamin D deficiency leads to as much as a 60 percent increase in cancer rates. Oncologists in Toronto, however, have been telling my cancer patients that they should take no supplemental vitamins when receiving radiation or chemotherapy. The reasons for this are nebulous, having no basis in scientific fact.

CHILDREN AND VITAMIN D DEFICIENCY

It may surprise you to know that seven out of ten children in the United States have been found to be deficient in vitamin D. So says a study reported August 4, 2009, by researchers at Albert Einstein College of Medicine of Yeshiva University. This finding means that millions of children could be at risk for cancer, diabetes, heart disease, and high blood pressure. This figure of 70 percent is similar to what I see in my practice whenever I order vitamin D blood tests on children ages four through twelve. Regardless of how good their diets may be, the vitamin D blood levels are often very low.

Study leader Michael Melamed was quoted as saying, "Several small studies had found a high prevalence of vitamin D deficiency in specific populations, but no one had examined this issue nationwide." A second researcher, Juhi Kumar, also was quoted as saying, "We expected the prevalence of vitamin D deficiency would be high, but the magnitude of the problem nationwide was shocking."

Both authors, therefore, have recommended that pediatricians routinely screen high-risk children for vitamin D deficiency and that parents ensure their kids get enough of the vitamin through a combination of sunshine and diet. Melamed advises, "It would be good for them to turn off the TV and send their kids outside. Just fifteen to twenty minutes a day should be enough. And unless they burn easily, don't put sunscreen on them until they've been out in the sun for ten minutes, so they get the good stuff but not sun damage."

Curiously enough, most pediatricians in the Toronto area pay no attention to this significant risk factor for all disease. In fact, I have yet to see a pediatrician in Toronto even order a vitamin D blood test for a patient. This is a personal clinical observation based on reports from parents who have taken their children to pediatricians. Having often been admonished in the past by pediatricians for prescribing vitamins, I now consider it my turn to admonish them for overlooking such important data.

In 2008, researchers at Moores Cancer Center at the University of California, San Diego, reported that six hundred thousand cases of cancer worldwide could be prevented each year by increasing the blood levels of vitamin D. These researchers found an inverse association between serum vitamin D levels and the risk of cancer. The more vitamin D, the lower the risk. Sixteen different types of cancer can be prevented by higher levels of vitamin D. These include breast, colon, lung, ovarian, pancreatic, and prostate cancers.

A patient in my practice who had been taking large doses of vitamin D and other natural remedies as part of her regimen against non-Hodgkin's lymphoma recently visited her oncologist, who queried her about what she was doing that cleared up her cancer. After all, she had not been getting either chemotherapy or radiation, and the numerous tumors had completely disappeared over a period of six months. The patient sheepishly replied that all she was doing was taking vitamins, minerals, and herbs. "Oh, spontaneous remission," remarked the oncologist.

Cancer specialists still truly believe that any cancer that gets better with natural remedies could only have come about by "spontaneous remission." That's just another way of saying that the disease went away only because of an act of God or the mysterious powers of the human mind. Vitamins, apparently, had nothing to do with it. Remind me to ask an oncologist sometime why so many patients in my practice experience this "spontaneous remission." I'm seeing it daily.

Could cancer be prevented or treated effectively by boosting the blood levels of vitamin D? I do not want readers to think that vitamin D is the answer to cancer, but I do want everyone to consider it an integral part of the solution. Don't start with any cancer treatment without knowing that your vitamin D blood level is at an optimal concentration, and don't be bashful about asking your doctor for blood testing.

A great deal of new research proves that vitamin D—whether from sun exposure, a sunlamp, or an oral supplement—can be of tremendous help for any cancer patient. The bare minimum amount of vitamin D that we should all be consuming is at least ten times higher than what has previously been recommended by most health authorities. Exactly how much daily is needed to prevent cancer is not yet known, but current estimates are in the 5,000–10,000 IU range.

BREAST-FEEDING

Breast-feeding may be the only source of vitamin D for some infants or toddlers. A 1998 study done in a Texas hospital analyzed cases of rickets and found that all the children were either African American or Hispanic and were consequently dark-skinned. You will recall that dark-skinned individuals are more prone to vitamin D deficiency because of the UVB-blocking effect of the dark pigment (melanin) in their skin. Consequently, these children—who were fed only breast milk by mothers with vitamin D deficiency—were much more likely to develop rickets than their Caucasian counterparts. It is therefore recommended that infants and toddlers of color receive vitamin D supplements, even if they live in a southern climate most of the year.

Vitamin D deficiency leads to as much as a 60 percent increase in cancer rates.

Breast Cancer

Breast cancer is the most common cancer in the Western world. The effect of vitamin D on breast cancer has received a great deal of attention ever since 1989 when a British medical journal, *The Lancet*, reported the regression of breast tumors with vitamin D supplementation in an animal model. In humans, it has been established that women living in the sunniest regions are three times less likely to develop breast cancer than those living in regions without as much sun.

In 1997, British researchers found that women with breast cancer and the highest blood levels of vitamin D had the best prognosis. The lower the blood level of vitamin D, the more rapid the fatal outcome of the disease. Vitamin D appears to retard breast cancer by regulating cell cycles and forcing apoptosis (cancer cell death). In other words, it works very much like some chemotherapy agents. The pharmaceutical industry has attempted to take advantage of this fact by manufacturing and experimenting with synthetic vitamin D analogues. Vitamin D cannot be patented. Consequently, drug companies could not make huge profits on a naturally occurring nutrient or hormone.

Unfortunately, while all these drug analogues worked well in the test tube to destroy cancer cells, in the human body they caused vitamin D toxicity in the form of dangerously high blood calcium levels. Synthetic lookalikes do not work like the real deal.

Vitamin D and calcium supplementation also seems to reduce any abnormality found on a routine mammogram. So said a 2004 Canadian study that indicated that women adequately nourished in vitamin D had one-fourth the number of abnormalities on mammograms.

Vitamin D works very much like some chemotherapy agents.

Colorectal Cancer

Colorectal cancer is the second most common cancer in the Western world. While many factors contribute to this type of cancer, vitamin D deficiency is thought to play a major role. The connection between colorectal cancer incidence and vitamin D deficiency was first noted in 1980 by Cedric Garland and his brother Frank Garland of the University of California at San Diego. They reported that death from the disease was less likely to occur in those who lived in sunny climates. In 1985, their study following 2,100 men for nineteen years indicated that the colon cancer rate was twice as high in those who consumed the least amount of vitamin D and calcium.

In 1989, the Garland brothers published a paper concluding that both breast and colon cancer were highest in cities with reduced sunlight caused by air pollution. They also found colon cancer rates to be four to six times higher in northern Europe and North American countries than in those countries closer to the equator.

Also in 1989, the Garlands made a similar correlation between vitamin D blood levels and colon cancer. They discovered that if blood levels of vitamin D were between 33 and 41 ng/ml, an individual was five times less likely to develop colon cancer. Other studies confirmed these findings. Raising the blood levels of vitamin D via sunshine exposure, eating more vitamin D–containing foods, or taking vitamin D supplements all had the same beneficial outcomes.

Prostate Cancer

Over thirty thousand deaths are caused by prostate cancer in North America each year, making it the second leading cause of cancer deaths in men. Its incidence is the leading cancer among men. There is a fair amount of evidence for a role of vitamin D in this disease. For example, in 1990 at the University of North Carolina at Chapel Hill, professor and researcher Gary Schwartz proposed a direct causal relationship between vitamin D deficiency and prostate cancer. Death from prostate cancer inversely correlates with the degree of ultraviolet irradiation, or sun exposure, the main source of vitamin D.

In 1992, Schwartz and colleague Carol Hanchette observed that American men were ten times more likely to develop prostate cancer than Japanese men who were consuming much higher amounts of vitamin D due to their intakes of fatty fish. Japanese men also consume higher amounts of soy products and omega-3 fatty acids than their American counterparts. Omega-3 fatty acids protect against the destruction of vitamin D, which can be destroyed in the body by chemicals, drugs, and pollutants. In people who are deficient in omega-3 fatty acids, vitamin D reserves are lower, and supplementation may have to be higher.

Omega-3 fatty acids protect against the destruction of vitamin D, which can be destroyed in the body by chemicals, drugs, and pollutants.

Research over the past two decades has consistently showed that men who received more sunlight were less likely to die from prostate cancer. The proof that vitamin D was the responsible factor came in a 1993 study by Roman Skowronski and colleagues. They discovered that prostate cancer cell lines all possessed a vitamin D receptor and that vitamin D "dramatically inhibited" the growth of the cell lines. In 1995, Gary Miller and colleagues reported similar findings. The more vitamin D receptors found in a prostate cancer cell line, the greater the cancer inhibition produced by vitamin D.

In 2000, Merja Ahonen and colleagues found a strong correlation between low blood levels of vitamin D and the development of prostate cancer. If blood levels were below 40 ng/ml, men were three times more likely to get prostate cancer and six times more likely to develop invasive cancers.

In 2001, Christopher Luscombe and his colleagues in England found that cumulative outdoor ultraviolet light exposure reduced the risk of advanced-stage prostate cancer. They also found that a history of many childhood sunburns dramatically reduced the risk of later-life prostate cancer. These studies, however, have not been able to convince mainstream dermatologists to change their advice about sunscreens and avoidance of sun exposure.

In 2003, Boston University researchers Tai Chen and Michael Holick concluded, "Adequate exposure to sunlight or oral supplementation might provide a simple way to increase synthesis of calcitriol (activated vitamin D) in the prostate and, therefore, decrease the risk of prostate cancer." They added, "Adequate vitamin D nutrition should be maintained, not only for bone health in men and women but because it might decrease the risk of prostate cancer and mitigate metastatic disease should it develop."

Finally, in 2004, Rheinhold Vieth and colleagues at the University of Toronto showed that taking 2,000 IU of vitamin D_3 reduced or prevented further increases in prostate-specific antigen (PSA) in the majority of men with advanced prostate cancer. This was the first report of a human-intervention trial that indicated that vitamin D_3 was effective in fighting cancer.

Taking 2,000 IU of vitamin D_3 reduced or prevented further increases in prostate-specific antigen (PSA) in the majority of men with advanced prostate cancer.

Pancreatic Cancer

About thirty thousand cases of pancreatic cancer are diagnosed in the United States each year. Since successful treatment of the disease is relatively rare, knowing how to prevent the disease would certainly be welcomed.

A 2006 published study led by researchers at Northwestern and Harvard Universities found that one could reduce the risk of getting pancreatic cancer by as much as 43 percent simply by supplementing with a mere 400 IU of vitamin D daily. According to Northwestern University researcher Halycon Skinner, "In concert with laboratory results suggesting antitumor effects of vitamin D, our results point to a possible role for vitamin D in the prevention and possible reduction in mortality of pancreatic cancer. Since no other environmental or dietary factor showed this risk relationship, more study of vitamin D's role is warranted." The exact mechanism by which vitamin D works to prevent pancreatic cancer is unknown, but research in the coming years will undoubtedly reveal this to us.

CARDIOVASCULAR DISEASES

When optimal levels exist in the bloodstream, Vitamin D prevents hardening of the arteries. Also referred to as atherosclerosis, this generalized arterial disease is caused by calcium deposits. Extremely high or low blood levels of vitamin D causes calcification of the arteries. Calcification from an overdose of vitamin D requires many hundreds of thousands of international units and is very rare, whereas vitamin D deficiency is common and calcified arteries can be a direct result of this deficiency.

Conventional doctors often focus their attention on lowering cholesterol to prevent artery blockages that can cause heart attacks. Cholesterol levels have very little to do with it. In addition, it is now an established fact that heart disease is often triggered and perpetuated by inflammation, and vitamin D is an anti-inflammatory.

Cholesterol: The Good Stuff

Cholesterol has become unfairly synonymous with disease and death. Cholesterol is an integral part of the structure of every cell in the body, including the cells of all your blood vessels.

Cholesterol is a healing, or repairing, agent, and the body makes more of it as a response to oxidant stress from numerous sources. For example, if you smoke cigarettes, your cholesterol level is likely to be high because the body needs protection against the toxins found in tobacco smoke.

Life would cease to exist without cholesterol. The body uses cholesterol to manufacture cortisol, DHEA, estrogen, progesterone, and testosterone. Low levels of cholesterol could lead to deficiencies in these hormones and subsequent acceleration of aging.

Cholesterol insulates nerves and is responsible for a healthy nervous system. Many diseases of the brain and nervous system could be aggravated, if not caused by, low cholesterol levels. Approximately one-quarter of all the cholesterol in the body is found in the brain. The myelin sheath that covers every nerve in the body is at least one-fifth cholesterol. The communication between nerves and the integrity of messages between neurons is partially dependent on adequate cholesterol levels. The brain functions abnormally without sufficient cholesterol because receptors for serotonin require cholesterol to work properly. When cholesterol is limited, depression, memory impairment, suicide, and violence are all more likely to occur.

Cholesterol deficiency could lead to numerous digestive problems because bile salts are made in the liver from cholesterol, and bile salts are important for proper digestion. The body also manufactures vitamin D from cholesterol and, if cholesterol levels are low, a vitamin D deficiency could result. As we now know, low levels of vitamin D can increase the risk of getting cancer by as much as 60 percent. Could this be one of the mechanisms by which statin drugs increase cancer incidence? Low levels of vitamin D have been proven to weaken immunity. Consequently, lowering cholesterol could, in fact, be related to a greater death risk, especially from cancer.

Lowering cholesterol could, in fact, be related to a greater death risk, especially from cancer.

Cholesterol and Heart Attacks

It has never been conclusively shown that lowering cholesterol levels saves lives. Certainly, its efficacy in preventing a first heart attack is unproven. Half of all heart attacks occur with cholesterol levels well within the normal range. This "normal" range has changed frequently over the past thirty years, going lower and lower, thus making it seem that just about everyone's cholesterol level is too high.

Since the correlation between total cholesterol and heart disease is practically nonexistent, a stronger correlation was sought many years ago. Hence the myth of a "good" (HDL, or high-density lipoprotein) and a "bad" (LDL, or low-density lipoprotein) cholesterol was created. The truth is that cholesterol is just cholesterol. In the blood, it combines with other substances, like proteins, simply because fat and water do not mix well and proteins are good carriers of fat molecules.

The real cause of heart disease of almost any type is inflammation and not cholesterol levels. Where the inflammation comes from is the subject of great debate, but there is growing evidence for an infectious disease.

We are now being told more and more by big pharmaceutical companies that statin drugs (such as Crestor, Lescol, Lipitor, Mevacor, Pravachol, and Zocor) are also anti-inflammatory and that the real reason they work in preventing heart disease is through their anti-inflammatory effect. Bromelain, curcumin, digestive enzymes like pancreatin, vitamins C, D, and E, and many other natural remedies are also anti-inflammatory and can be obtained at a significantly lower cost. Furthermore, none carry the side effects seen with the statins.

We are all exposed to toxins from food, water, and air on a regular basis. The greater the toxin exposure, the more the body needs to protect itself. One way this occurs is with the production of more cholesterol by the liver. Suppress that function with a statin and you risk developing degenerative diseases more easily.

WHERE DOES CHOLESTEROL COME FROM?

At least 85 percent of the cholesterol in your blood comes from your liver, which manufactures it. If you consume high-cholesterol foods, your cholesterol blood levels temporarily increase. The liver then manufactures less cholesterol, and blood levels eventually decrease. If you eliminate cholesterol entirely from your diet, the liver will manufacture more of it.

Cholesterol blood levels can change significantly from one time of the day to another. In northern latitudes (above 40 degrees north), higher levels of cholesterol are seen in winter than in summer, possibly because of the cholesterol-lowering effect of the vitamin D we receive from sunshine during the summer. Cholesterol levels increase after an injury or surgery, and as a response to mental stress, an infection, or during and after a heart attack.

The real cause of heart disease of almost any type is inflammation and not cholesterol levels.

High Blood Pressure

Many studies now link sunlight exposure to the lowering of high blood pressure. Sunlight not only elevates vitamin D but also causes the release of chemicals called endorphins in the brain. These chemicals can reduce pain, induce relaxation, and lower blood pressure. In addition, vitamin D helps to control blood pressure and prevent stroke. The higher the vitamin D blood levels, the lower the blood pressure, and consequently the lower the incidence of stroke.

Emerging evidence has compared the blood pressure–lowering effects of vitamin D to angiotensin-converting enzyme (ACE) inhibitors, a class of blood pressure–lowering drugs commonly prescribed by conventional doctors. Don't go off your blood pressure pills yet, but do consider high-dose supplements of vitamin D and get your blood levels checked along with your blood pressure.

The higher the vitamin D blood levels, the lower the blood pressure, and consequently the lower the incidence of stroke.

Congestive Heart Failure

In 2006, a clinical trial published in the *American Journal of Clinical Nutrition* concluded that high doses of vitamin D could help people suffering from congestive heart failure (CHF). Conventional medicine usually treats this disease with diuretics like furosemide, heart stimulants like digitalis, and assorted heart rhythm medications.

Many factors are known to contribute to CHF. Recent research indicates that it may have something to do with the presence of inflammation. It is well known that high doses of vitamin D are anti-inflammatory, and this could explain its effectiveness in treating CHF. The dose used in the study was 2,000 IU per day, and the reduction in inflammatory factors in the blood was 43 percent compared with a placebo. Conceivably, higher, more adequate doses of vitamin D would have produced even more impressive numbers.

COENZYME Q10 BOOSTS HEART HEALTH

Coenzyme Q10 (CoQ10) is the most important nutrient for ideal heart function. It is used by the energy-producing cell organelles known as mitochondria and is vitally important for a normal cardiac output. Studies indicate that supplementing with coenzyme Q10 improves every measure of cardiac function. Three months of coenzyme Q10 supplementation can lower blood pressure in at least half the people who have elevated blood pressure. It has also been shown to be important in cancer treatment (especially in breast cancer), Parkinson's disease, and periodontal disease.

If you take drugs to lower cholesterol, you should be aware that statins like Crestor, Lipitor, Mevacor, Pravachol, and Zocor deplete coenzyme Q10 levels by at least 40 percent over a period of a year, creating such unwanted symptoms as fatigue, weak and tired muscles, lethargy, and a general sense of low energy. A deficiency of coenzyme Q10 can result in high blood pressure. Therefore, statins can theoretically increase your risk of having a heart attack or stroke.

Interestingly, one study done in 2009 indicates that 92 percent of people who developed muscle damage from statins (myositis-myalgia) were able to reverse this side effect with vitamin D supplementation. The take-away message here is that if you are on a statin, take a coenzyme Q10 supplement but also get your vitamin D blood levels checked.

AUTOIMMUNE DISEASES

More than one hundred different diseases have been classified as autoimmune. Colitis, multiple sclerosis, psoriasis, rheumatoid arthritis, scleroderma, systemic lupus erythematosus, and thyroiditis are among the better known.

An autoimmune disease manifests when the body's own immune system attacks various organs, resulting in inflammation in that organ. The cause of most autoimmune diseases is said to be unknown, but most have been related to toxins like mercury as well as deficiencies. There is also evidence that unsuspected food allergies (especially to gluten and dairy products) may be involved. The most important but overlooked cause, however, may well be vitamin D deficiency.

People sometimes die as a result of these chronic diseases. The treatments for them can be quite toxic, especially when immunosuppressive drugs like methotrexate, Plaquenil (hydroxychloroquine), prednisone, and Remicade (infliximab) are used. A few lucky individuals can get away with controlling their autoimmune disease with nonsteroidal anti-inflammatory drugs (NSAIDs), but even these have significant side effects that include gastrointestinal bleeding and heart attacks. Some would even say that the treatments are more toxic than the disease.

Decades before we knew of the anti-inflammatory benefits of vitamin D, Dale Alexander wrote books and spoke enthusiastically about healing miracles associated with the use of cod liver oil. Although he lacked a professional science background, Dale Alexander was known as the "codfather" and popularized the use of cod liver oil around the world. As you know, cod liver oil is rich in vitamin D.

If you look at people who suffer from one of the many autoimmune diseases, you are likely to find that their blood levels of vitamin D are low or close to being low in the vast majority of cases. Certainly, I have witnessed this phenomenon for years in the blood test results of patients in my private practice.

If you examine published medical studies on autoimmune diseases like rheumatoid arthritis and lupus, you are likely to see that these diseases and their severity are inversely correlated with blood levels of vitamin D. In other words, if you have an autoimmune disease, you may well be vitamin D deficient and your disease could conceivably be reversed with vitamin D supplementation.

VITAMIN D AND AUTOIMMUNE DISEASES

If you are plagued by any of these autoimmune diseases, vitamin D supplementation may make all the difference in the world for you.

achlorhydria

Addison's disease

alopecia areata

amyotrophic lateral sclerosis (ALS, Lou Gehrig's disease)

ankylosing spondylitis

anti-GBM nephritis or anti-TBM nephritis

antiphospholipid syndrome (Hughes syndrome)

aplastic anemia

arthritis

asthma

atopic allergy

atopic dermatitis

autoimmune chronic active hepatitis

autoimmune inner ear disease (AIED)

autoimmune lymphoproliferative syndrome (ALPS)

Balo disease

Behçet's disease

bullous pemphigoid

cardiomyopathy

celiac disease

chronic fatigue immune dysfunction syndrome (CFIDS)

Churg-Strauss syndrome

cicatricial pemphigoid

Cogan's syndrome

cold agglutinin disease

colitis

cranial arteritis

CREST syndrome

Crohn's disease

Cushing's syndrome

Degos disease (malignant atrophic papulosis)

dermatitis

dermatomyositis

Devic's disease

diabetes, Type 1

diabetes, Type 2

Dressler's syndrome

discoid lupus erythematosus (DLE)

eczema

eosinophilic fasciitis

epidermolysis bullosa acquisita

essential mixed cryoglobulinemia

Evans' syndrome

fibromyalgia (fibromyositis)

fibrosing alveolitis

gastritis

giant cell arteritis

glomerulonephritis

Goodpasture's disease

Graves' disease
Guillain-Barré syndrome (GBS)
Hashimoto's thyroiditis
hemolytic anemia
Henoch-Schönlein purpura (HSPP)
hepatitis
idiopathic adrenal atrophy
idiopathic pulmonary fibrosis
idiopathic thrombocytopenic purpura
IgA nephropathy (Berger's disease)
inflammatory demyelinating polyneuropathy
irritable bowel syndrome
Kawasaki disease
lichen planus (LP)
lupoid hepatitis
lupus
Lyme disease
Ménière's disease
mixed connective tissue disease
multiple myeloma
multiple sclerosis
myasthenia gravis
myositis
ocular cicatricial pemphigoid
osteoporosis
pars planitis
pemphigus vulgaris
polyglandular autoimmune syndromes
polymyalgia rheumatica (PMR)
polymyositis
primary biliary cirrhosis
primary sclerosing cholangitis (PSC)
psoriasis
Raynaud's phenomenon
Reiter's syndrome
rheumatic fever
rheumatoid arthritis
sarcoidosis
scleritis
scleroderma
Sjögren's syndrome
sticky blood syndrome
stiff-man syndrome
Still's disease
sydenham chorea (SD)
systemic lupus erythematosus (SLE)
Takayasu's arteritis
temporal arteritis
ulcerative colitis
vasculitis
vitiligo
Wegener's granulomatosis
Wilson's syndrome

We now know that the vitamin D content of cod liver oil provides amazing healing of arthritis and about one hundred other inflammatory diseases. When combined with omega-3 fatty acids, vitamin D reduces inflammation without the toxicity seen with immunosuppressant drugs, steroid drugs like prednisone, and NSAIDs.

When combined with omega-3 fatty acids, vitamin D reduces inflammation without the toxicity seen with immunosuppressant drugs, steroid drugs like prednisone, and NSAIDs.

Multiple Sclerosis

For years, epidemiological studies have suggested that vitamin D deficiency may somehow be involved as a cause of multiple sclerosis (MS) simply because the incidence as well as the severity of the disease are reduced in areas of the world where people have more or longer exposure to sunshine. This kind of data has been so striking that people with MS have taken it upon themselves to supplement with high doses of vitamin D without medical approval. Fortunately, due to the high safety profile of vitamin D, and because very recent studies have proved that vitamin D is beneficial for MS, these people have been very successful in either preventing MS attacks or reducing the severity of their symptoms.

One study done in 2007 by researcher Samantha Kimball and colleagues at the University of Toronto indicated that MS lesions seen on brain scans were reduced by more than half with vitamin D supplementation. Usually, doses of 8,000–10,000 IU daily are required, but regular blood testing to make sure the 25-hydroxy vitamin D levels are between 100–250 ng/ml can indicate whether MS patients need slightly more or less than that dose. Certainly, careful sun exposure is one thing that should be strongly entertained.

Some very good news has come out for families with a history of MS. It seems that vitamin D adequacy may be necessary to prevent the expression of a gene that is thought to code for MS. According to the study leader, Sreeram Ramagopalan, a postdoctoral fellow at the University of Oxford: "Our study implies that taking vitamin D supplements during pregnancy and the early years may reduce the risk of a child developing MS in later life." The February 2009 study was published in the *Public Library of Science Genetics Journal* reports (see www.plos.org).

One would hope that such findings encourage mainstream doctors to promote vitamin D supplementation for not only MS but also autoimmune diseases of all kinds: cancer, chronic fatigue syndrome, fibromyalgia, and numerous other chronic diseases that respond well to supplementation. However, there is a prejudice against vitamin therapy in mainstream medicine, and the fact that vitamin D has proved effective against these diseases may make mainstream doctors anxious because they usually prescribe toxic pharmaceuticals like corticosteroids, immunosuppressants, and nonsteroidal anti-inflammatory drugs. They typically do not prescribe vitamin D, and if they do, the doses are far too low to be effective.

Vitamin D deficiency may be involved as a cause of multiple sclerosis because the incidence as well as the severity of the disease are reduced in areas of the world where people have more or longer exposures to sunshine.

Thyroid Autoantibodies (Autoimmune Thyroiditis)

Many people with borderline or even conclusive thyroid disease have elevated antibodies against their own thyroid gland. Technically, this is called autoimmune thyroiditis and can lead to both over- and underactive thyroid disease. The mineral selenium (200–400 mcg daily) will lower or eliminate the antibodies in many cases. When the problem persists, high-dose vitamin D supplements (10,000–20,000 IU daily) will work to reduce or eliminate the autoantibodies. As with any autoimmune disease, it is wise to determine whether vitamin D is at an optimal level.

OTHER HEALTH CONDITIONS

Acne

Most people who suffer from acne have noticed that exposure to sunshine improves the condition substantially and that acne seems to be reduced in general during the summer months. This may well be due to the fact that with greater sun exposure, the blood levels of vitamin D increase. In fact, it was known as far back as 1938 that vitamin D supplementation would help reduce and eliminate acne.

Vitamin D is, after all, a hormone. It is a well-known fact that acne is regulated to a large extent by hormone balance. Balancing hormones is one of the major functions of vitamin D, and it's something that involves all the glandular systems in the body.

Here's what John Cannell of the Vitamin D Council said in one of his newsletters: "I have had some reports that vitamin D cured acne but, frankly, I didn't believe them. Then I ran across this 1938 paper. You can read the entire paper yourself and see what 5,000–14,000 IU per day did for these patients with severe acne. . . . Of the 132 acne patients studied, 28 percent were 'much better' at three months and 47 percent were 'healed' at three months."

Aging

Can optimal levels of vitamin D retard aging? One recent medical journal reports that it may be a distinct possibility. The November 2007 edition of the *American Journal of Clinical Nutrition* describes an association between longer chromosome telomeres and increased levels of vitamin D. Telomeres are caps at the ends of chromosomes that shorten with age as well as with oxidative stress and inflammation. The shorter the telomere, the more aging is seen to occur. The longer the telomere, the greater the delay in age-related diseases.

The study found lower levels of oxidative stress and inflammation and longer telomeres in people with higher vitamin D blood levels. The reason for this is that vitamin D decreases inflammation.

Alzheimer's Disease and Dementia

Alzheimer's disease is the most common form of dementia and affects over thirteen million people worldwide. Vitamin D receptors exist in the brain, spinal cord, and central nervous system. A growing number of studies demonstrate very strong links between low blood levels of vitamin D and the presence of the signs and symptoms of Alzheimer's disease and different forms of dementia. The lower the vitamin D blood level, the worse the performance on cognitive tests. Moreover, adding supplemental vitamin D to the diet or providing increased sunlight exposure not only improves the blood levels of vitamin D but also the cognitive function in those suffering from these forms of brain degeneration. The belief by most scientists at this time is that vitamin D somehow enhances important brain chemicals and protects brain cells from deterioration.

It has been known for quite some time that Alzheimer's victims have an increased risk of hip fractures. Vitamin D deficiency is more common in older adults and so is the incidence of neurological and psychiatric illness. In one study done in 2006, 58 percent of the participants age fifty and older were found to have low blood levels of vitamin D (defined as less than 20 ng/ml). The average vitamin D level in the group was 18.58 ng/ml, a far cry from the optimum levels. These people were found to have an 88 percent higher chance of suffering from anxiety or depression, and they performed worse on mental-function tests than those with more optimal vitamin D levels. There is no question that vitamin D deficiency can be associated with suboptimal brain health, and studies do show substantial improvements in cognitive function or performance when high-dose vitamin D is given.

A growing number of studies demonstrate very strong links between low blood levels of vitamin D and the presence of the signs and symptoms of Alzheimer's disease and different forms of dementia.

Asthma

An estimated 20 million people in the United States suffer from asthma. Its incidence has increased by more than 300 percent in just the last two decades. Asthma attacks can be linked to low blood levels of vitamin D. Massive doses of vitamin D in the neighborhood of 50,000–150,000 IU daily for three days have reduced wheezing and coughing without the use of the typical asthma drugs and steroid inhalers. This is well worth trying for those who have asthma but should only be done with medical supervision, considering the toxicity of steroids and other drugs.

A recent study involving six hundred children with asthma showed that the severity of the disease was inversely correlated with the blood levels of vitamin D. In other words, the lower the vitamin D blood level, the worse the asthma. In addition, the lower the vitamin D, the worse the allergies, the higher the levels of immunoglobulin E (IgE) and eosinophils (two markers for allergy severity), and the higher the likelihood of hospitalization for asthma.

A 2007 study from the *Journal of Allergy and Clinical Immunology* concluded these three points:

1. Vitamin D has been linked to immune system and lung development *in utero*, and our epidemiologic studies show that higher vitamin D intake by pregnant women reduces asthma risk by as much as 40 percent in children three to five years old.
2. Providing adequate vitamin D supplementation during pregnancy may lead to significant decreases in asthma incidence in young children.
3. *In vitro* evidence supports our contention that vitamin D insufficiency may worsen asthma severity, and we suspect that giving vitamin D supplements to asthma patients who are deficient may help with their asthma control.

The good news is that you can safely take high doses of vitamin D even if you are on prescription steroid inhalers or other antiwheezing drugs. You should be able to either cut down or eliminate these drugs through the use of vitamin D. Just make sure you get your vitamin D blood levels checked at regular intervals.

Athletic Performance

According to the Vitamin D Council's John Cannell, "Steroid hormones are substances made from cholesterol that circulate in your body and work at distant sites by setting in motion genetic protein transcription. That is, both vitamin D and testosterone set in motion your genome, the stuff of life. While testosterone is a sex steroid hormone, vitamin D is a pleomorphic steroid hormone." ("Pleomorphic" means it can assume different forms.)

Many performance-enhancing drugs and food supplements are banned from athletic competitions. Presently, vitamin D is allowed and may make a big difference in the performance of many athletes. In the 1960s and '70s, when German and Russian athletes seemed to win just about every Olympic medal, Germany and Russia coincidentally published the most convincing studies in their medical journals on the athletic performance–enhancing effects of vitamin D. Vitamin D supplementation will definitely improve athletic performance in vitamin D–deficient people (which is just about everyone, it seems). Studies do show that taking vitamin D will make you faster, stronger, better coordinated, and mentally tougher as an athlete.

A 2009 study by Kate Ward, a researcher at England's University of Manchester, found that vitamin D helped young teenaged girls jump higher. Vitamin D supplementation increases the number and size of fast-twitch muscle fibers, which are needed for optimal performance at physical activities such as sprinting and weight lifting. To achieve improved athletic performance, your vitamin D blood levels must be at least 75 ng/ml. Get your blood levels checked.

Autism

Autism, or autistic spectrum disorder (ASD), is a poorly understood phenomenon of the twenty-first century. It is characterized by poor social and verbal functioning and repetitive or stereotyped behaviors. There are varying degrees of childhood developmental delays, and some of the odd behaviors can be self-damaging.

Childhood autism is increasing at a rate of more than 20 percent per year in North America. One recent study argues that incidence of the disorder has risen thirtyfold in a seven-year period. A British study in 2006 concluded that one in eighty-six children will develop the disorder. These numbers are epidemic in nature. Some experts have blamed this alarmingly high incidence on mercury in vaccines and the fact that children are receiving more vaccines than ever, but the scientists at the Vitamin D Council have another plausible theory: the miniscule amounts of vitamin D in prenatal supplements are simply not enough to provide the fetal brain's very thirsty vitamin D receptors. The developing brain, with its plentiful vitamin D receptors, is deprived, and vitamin D deprivation leads to brain damage.

The National Institutes of Mental Health have also gone on record as stating that it is vital for expectant mothers to get adequate amounts of vitamin D so the baby's brain can develop and function normally. There is considerable evidence that vitamin D is required by the developing brain. For example, French researchers have found that vitamin D deficiency disrupts thirty-six important brain proteins during fetal development. Brain enlargement and enlargement of the brain's fluid-filled ventricles are also seen with vitamin D deficiency, and these are two characteristics common to autistic children.

Brain inflammation is something that dramatically affects cognitive performance. There is evidence of inflammation in the autistic brain, and it is well established that vitamin D has strong anti-inflammatory properties.

The Vitamin D Council argues for aggressive vitamin D supplementation for autistic children. The starting dose recommended for these unfortunate children is 5,000 IU daily. Blood tests for 25-hydroxy vitamin D should be checked monthly and the vitamin D doses adjusted appropriately. To prevent autism, the Vitamin D Council also recommends that expectant mothers take 5,000 IU daily. I am one physician who strongly believes this advice, mainly based on the fact that virtually all pregnant women in my practice tend to have low levels of vitamin D on their initial blood tests.

One recent study indicates that autistic children have abnormal bones, which in turn indicates a genetic abnormality in vitamin D metabolism. While the use of vitamin D for autism is only at the theory stage, the use of vitamin D in these children is a low-risk intervention with a potentially happy outcome. Since most of the medical and conventional treatments for autism are so dismal, supplementing with vitamin D may be well worth a try. For parents who want more information on the connection between autism and vitamin D, there is an excellent review paper on this subject on the Life Extension website (www.lef.org).

There is considerable evidence that vitamin D is required by the developing brain.

The Common Cold and the Flu

At one period during Linus Pauling's lifetime, we were all convinced that the answer to the common cold was vitamin C. Although it is quite true that high doses of vitamin C reduce the severity and eliminate some of the more common symptoms of a cold, vitamin D appears to do a much better job of preventing this very common illness.

A very large 2009 study involving nineteen thousand American adults and adolescents has clearly shown that people with the lowest blood levels of vitamin D had significantly more recent cases of the common cold or the flu. Conversely, the higher the blood levels of vitamin D, the lower the rate of respiratory tract infections.

Adit Ginde of the University of Colorado at Denver and chief author of this study was quoted as saying, "The findings of our study support an important role for vitamin D in the prevention of common respiratory infections such as colds and the flu. Individuals with common lung diseases, such as asthma or emphysema, may be particularly susceptible to respiratory infections from vitamin D deficiency."

Influenza, commonly known as the flu, is a respiratory infection caused by a variety of viruses. Unlike the common cold, which is also a respiratory infection caused by viruses, the flu can cause fever, headache, and extreme exhaustion. Body aches, especially in the muscles, joints, and ligaments, can be severe enough to force complete bed rest. Other flu symptoms are chills, a dry cough, body aches, stuffy nose, and a sore throat.

It is estimated that at least fifty million people in North America get the flu each season (November to March). Children are two to three times more likely than adults to get sick with the flu. More than one hundred thousand people are hospitalized and at least twenty thousand die from the flu and its complications every year.

Many consider the flu an inevitable fact of winter, but this is not necessarily the case. Although our lifestyles may not always allow it, the best way to prevent this viral illness is to keep our health at its optimum. This can be done by getting enough rest, limiting stress, and by eating a nutritious diet.

One way of maintaining good health is to ensure the body has an adequate supply of vitamins and minerals. Nutrient requirements vary from one individual to the next, but any formula for the immune system should contain beta-carotene (provitamin A); vitamins A, B_6, C, and D; and zinc.

Ever wonder why some people are more prone to colds and flus? One study indicates that the incidence of upper respiratory tract infections is inversely correlated with vitamin D blood levels. Simply put, the lower the vitamin D blood level, the higher the likelihood of infection. This is also an observation I have made on numerous occasions with my private-practice patients. Each year I see infection rates rise in the winter as vitamin D levels plummet, and each summer the exact opposite occurs.

John Cannell of the Vitamin D Council suggests that high-dose vitamin D (50,000 IU) be consumed for three days at the first sign of a cold or the flu. Vitamin D protects us from the cold and flu in other ways. Vitamin D supports the immune system, prevents inflammation, and increases white blood cell activity to protect the lungs from infection.

People with the lowest blood levels of vitamin D had significantly more recent cases of the common cold or the flu.

Should You Get the Flu Shot?

My advice is to rethink that annual flu shot. Aside from the fact that there have been a number of very good scientific studies proving that the flu shot is no better than a placebo, vitamin D appears to be far more important. Vitamin D has strong antibiotic properties, and some studies indicate that optimal blood levels will prevent the flu much better than flu shots.

Proponents of the flu vaccine boast a 70 percent effectiveness rate, but clinical experience proves otherwise. For example, in British Columbia in 2000, it was reported that of thirty-two individuals in a nursing home who received a flu shot, thirty had contracted the flu. That same year, nursing homes throughout British Columbia reported a much higher death rate from the flu than what would be expected, despite a 100 percent vaccination rate.

A 1993 Dutch article reported that 50 percent of the vaccinated population in a home for the elderly caught the flu compared to 48 percent of the unvaccinated group. The excuse for such failures is that the wrong virus was predicted for use in the flu vaccine. The truth is that if the flu shot prevents the flu, it's purely on a placebo basis.

The actual composition of the flu vaccine is based on an educated guess made by a consensus of about thirty public-health experts. These "experts" meet annually with the U.S. Food and Drug Administration to predict which specific strains of influenza will invade the country in the coming year. If this sounds unscientific to you, it's because it is. At best, keeping in mind factors such as mistakes in production, transport, and storage, the flu vaccine's effectiveness rate is only about 20 percent. Placebo shots are at least 30 percent effective.

Beyond its very questionable effectiveness, the flu vaccine, consumed faithfully by the public without question each year, has a disturbing history of potential toxicity. The vaccine contains formaldehyde, a known cancer-causing agent. It also contains the preservative thimerosal, a derivative of mercury and a known neurotoxin linked to brain damage and autoimmune diseases. Aluminum is yet another flu-vaccine ingredient. When mercury is not in the vaccine, it is replaced by equivalent amounts of aluminum, which can eventually be deposited in the brain. Mercury and aluminum are two toxic heavy metals that have been associated with an increased incidence of Alzheimer's disease and, possibly, other neurodegenerative illnesses.

In 1976, 565 cases of Guillain-Barré syndrome (GBS) paralysis were reported along with other neurological problems and many unexplained deaths among recently vaccinated older adults. With only a 10 percent or less reporting of adverse vaccine reactions by doctors in both the United States and Canada, the true flu-vaccine damage figures are grossly underestimated. Vaccine manufacturers counter this concern by saying that today's vaccines do not carry the same risk of GBS. This may be true, but many cases of GBS as well as other neurological problems are still occurring after flu vaccines. Additionally, product inserts still state that individuals who have a history of GBS have a much greater likelihood of developing GBS after receiving the flu shot.

Other side effects reported with the flu vaccine are abnormal blood pressure, allergic asthma, ataxia, brachial plexus neuropathy, encephalitis, eye problems, fever, gastrointestinal problems, general malaise, hives, low platelet count, muscle pain, optic neuritis, other circulatory abnormalities, polyneuritis, respiratory tract infections, and systemic anaphylaxis. Those with a severe allergy to eggs are advised against the flu shot because of its chicken egg content.

Vitamin D has strong antibiotic properties, and some studies indicate that optimal blood levels will prevent the flu far better than flu shots.

Vitamin D and the Flu Study in Canada

Drug companies that are manufacturing the flu vaccine and flu medications may be somewhat dismayed by the August 10, 2009, announcement by the Public Health Agency of Canada (PHAC) that they will be investigating the role of vitamin D against the H1N1 virus (swine flu). In the United States, no such activity by any government agency has been announced.

Here is the announcement:

> Researchers in PHAC are working with colleagues at McMaster University and with partners at other universities and hospitals to determine whether there is a correlation between severe disease and low vitamin D levels and/or a person's genetic make up. This line of research in seasonal influenza will be adapted to H1N1.
>
> If we find that there is a correlation between severe disease and vitamin D levels we shall, with our partners in the future, conduct randomized controlled studies to determine whether vitamin D can be used as a means to mitigate severe seasonal influenza. PHAC intends to adapt this strategy to H1N1 in order to prevent severe outcomes of infection.

THE INFECTIOUS DISEASE SPECIALIST IS OUT

If you have an infection, the truth is that you need more vitamin D. Vitamin D acts as a natural antibiotic, working against every type of microbe (bacteria, fungi, parasites, viruses). That's why I think the following anecdote is so ironic. It demonstrates that even our brightest medical professionals may be unqware of this amazing property of vitamin D:

A middle-aged patient of mine recently phoned to ask me to give her a vaccine to prevent hepatitis. I told her that I do not stock the vaccine, nor do I believe in its merits. I referred her to a travel clinic headed by one of the top infectious disease specialists in Toronto, but when she phoned his office, the message on the tape was this: "I'm sorry but I cannot come to the phone right now. I'm sitting here looking out my window, quarantining myself and waiting to recover from the swine flu. I don't know when I'll be back, but rest assured I am well medicated and will be able to return your call sometime in the foreseeable future. If you need to see an infectious-disease specialist more urgently, see one of my associates."

No one has to wait for the results of this study before attempting to boost his or her own vitamin D levels. Cannell and many other researchers have already published numerous studies proving that supplementation of vitamin D can dramatically enhance immunity against virtually any infectious disease.

Crohn's Disease and Ulcerative Colitis

Crohn's disease and ulcerative colitis are often lumped together under the term "inflammatory bowel disease." They can cause life-impairing symptoms and even death, and are usually treated aggressively with powerful drugs by gastroenterologists (intestinal specialists). The major interventions in use today against IBD are corticosteroids like prednisone; antibiotics like Flagyl (metronidazole); aminosalicylates like Asacol, Azulfidine (sulfasalazine), or Pentasa (mesalamine); immunosuppressive drugs like cyclosporine and Imuran (azathioprine); and surgery to remove the diseased bowel. Unfortunately, the ultimate fate of some victims of ulcerative colitis is a total colectomy, which is curative but leaves the patient with an ileostomy (an artificial abdominal opening with a disposable pouch for stool collection). Special diets, nutritional supplements, and herbs are rarely, if ever, prescribed for those who suffer from these intestinal disorders, despite numerous reports of clinical successes using less toxic, natural approaches.

Both diseases involve bowel inflammation as well as inflammation of tissues outside the gut. There are differences between the two types of IBD, but there is also some degree of overlap with respect to signs and symptoms.

Crohn's disease (granulomatous ileitis or ileocolitis) is primarily a disease of white adults between the ages of twenty and forty, although it can occur in both children and the elderly. Its main signs and symptoms include an abdominal pain or mass, diarrhea, fever, weight loss, rectal bleeding, anal fissures, abscesses, and arthritis. In a minority of cases, there may be inflammation of the liver, kidney, and skin. The disease process involves only the small bowel in 30 percent of patients, only the colon in 15 percent, and both the small bowel and colon in 55 percent. The diagnosis is usually made by X-rays or a biopsy. Symptoms may include an increased urgency to defecate (up to ten to twenty times a day), bloody and watery bowel movements containing pus and mucus, normal or dry stools (constipation) if the disease is limited to the rectosigmoidal area, fever, general malaise, weight loss or anorexia, dehydration, joint pain, skin changes, liver disease, and eye problems.

Ulcerative colitis is a chronic inflammatory disease that deteriorates the lining of the large bowel. It shows up primarily in the twenty-to-forty age group and predominantly affects females. Most often, the inflammation begins at the rectum and extends up through the colon. The inflammation can progress until ulcerations and abscesses develop. In some patients, the disease can be mild and localized or excruciatingly painful with perforations of the colon. There is usually diarrhea, with blood and mucus in the stool. Sudden attacks followed by periods of remission are typical.

Ulcerative colitis tends to recur in families, and there is a high incidence of arthritis, ankylosing spondylitis, eczema, and hay fever coexisting with the bowel disorder. There is a school of thought that believes that inflammatory bowel disease, especially ulcerative colitis, is the result of an allergy or hypersensitivity reaction to certain foods by the colon. Some practitioners have observed an association between Crohn's disease and dental-amalgam mercury sensitivity, while others, like British gastroenterologist Andrew Wakefield, have recently associated Crohn's disease with the MMR (measles, mumps, rubella) vaccine.

Salicylate (aspirin) sensitivity can be found in some patients with ulcerative colitis. Some researchers have shown the existence of circulating antibodies against cow's milk and other foods, especially wheat and other grains. The foods that most often trigger ulcerative colitis are cow's milk, wheat, and yeast-containing foods. IBD has been reported to be directly connected to a diet high in junk food such as fried foods, high-fat snacks, processed foods, soda pop, sugar, and white-flour products.

In both Crohn's disease and ulcerative colitis, antifungal medications like colchicine, ketoconazole, and nystatin have been documented to reverse the inflammatory process in some cases. This and the many positive reports of disease reversal through the use of natural antifungal therapies support the theory that both Crohn's disease and ulcerative colitis have a strong connection to chronic fungal infection.

Another theory is based on studies showing that IBD is a form of exaggerated allergic response to the presence of intestinal bugs that healthier individuals who are genetically less susceptible tolerate without difficulty. Allergy desensitization techniques, nutritional programs designed to repair a "leaky gut," and the use of natural antibiotics, digestive enzymes, antifungals, and immune-system modulators may all play a role in reversing IBD naturally.

A variety of factors including heredity have been implicated as causing IBD, but it is generally believed to be an autoimmune disorder, one in which a person's immune system makes antibodies against his or her own gastrointestinal tract cells. A recent factor that may directly be involved in causing either of these autoimmune diseases is vitamin D deficiency.

Several studies have found low blood levels of vitamin D in those suffering from IBD, and patients from around the world have reported reversal of IBD signs and symptoms with vitamin D supplementation or increased sun exposure. Since many patients with Crohn's or colitis have trouble absorbing nutrients, including vitamin D, sun exposure or UVB light exposure might be more effective than using oral supplements. I recommend tanning beds or artificial ultraviolet light exposure in cases where the bowel fails to absorb vitamin D from an oral source. People who have had bowel surgery or suffer from bowel disease would benefit from using artificial ultraviolet light.

Several studies have found low blood levels of vitamin D in those suffering from IBD, and patients from around the world have reported reversal of IBD signs and symptoms with vitamin D supplementation or increased sun exposure.

Cystic Fibrosis

Cystic fibrosis (CF) affects approximately thirty thousand people in the United States. It is an inherited and fatal disease that causes victims to produce abnormally thick and sticky mucus that often obstructs the lung, leading to chronic bronchitis and other lung diseases. The mucus can also obstruct the pancreatic ducts and lead to abnormal digestion and chronic vitamin and mineral deficiencies. In 2005, average life expectancy for CF patients was thirty-three years.

About 25 percent of adults with CF have osteoporosis and about 40 percent have a less serious form of bone loss called osteopenia. In one recent study of adults with CF, it was found that over 80 percent had vitamin D deficiency. In this study, oral supplementation with 800,000 IU of vitamin D over eight weeks failed to correct the deficiency. The cause was probably due to malabsorption, a condition that is quite commonly associated with CF.

Depression

Psychiatrists should pay more attention to the mood-enhancing effects of vitamin D. Before 2000, many of the studies done on the effects of vitamin D on depression did not show any benefit, mostly because the daily dose used was only 400 IU. This is clearly inadequate. In 1999, however, Bruce Hollis, a leading vitamin D researcher at the Medical University of South Carolina, and associates found that 100,000 IU of vitamin D_3 given as a one-time oral dose improved depression symptoms better in patients suffering from seasonal affective disorder (SAD) than light therapy, the usual conventional treatment. Researchers have generally found that the lower the initial blood levels of 25-hydroxy vitamin D, the more likely vitamin D supplementation would improve symptoms of depression.

One of the reasons why vitamin D improves depression is that it controls an enzyme called tyrosine hydroxylase in the adrenal gland. This enzyme is needed for the production of dopamine, epinephrine, and norepinephrine. If these neurotransmitters are low, depression is often the result. Vitamin D deficiency is not the only cause of depression, but every person using antidepressant medicines should have a blood test for vitamin D levels.

Every person using antidepressant medicines should have a blood test for vitamin D levels.

Diabetes

Vitamin D appears to be needed for normal insulin secretion and glucose tolerance. There is growing evidence that both Type 1 and Type 2 diabetes can be prevented or outcomes improved by enhancing the blood levels of vitamin D.

In someone who has a low level of vitamin D, the pancreas synthesizes less insulin. Therefore, the lower the vitamin D in the blood, the lower the production of insulin. Cataracts, a complication of abnormally high sugar levels, are also preventable if blood levels of vitamin D remain high.

In 2003, the *American Journal of Clinical Nutrition* reported that the use of cod liver oil in the first year of life was associated with a significantly lower risk of Type 1 diabetes. In 2006, *Diabetes Care* concluded that vitamin D deficiency is more common in Type 2 diabetes than in Type 1 diabetes and is unrelated to age, gender, or insulin treatment.

If you have diabetes of either type or a strong family history of the disease, make sure to ask your doctor to check your blood levels of vitamin D along with routinely testing for blood sugar. With appropriate supplementation, you may well be able to prevent a long list of complications that usually occur with diabetes.

Vitamin D deficiency is more common in Type 2 diabetes than in Type 1 diabetes and is unrelated to age, gender, or insulin treatment.

Eczema

Eczema is one of the most common inflammatory skin problems for which individuals of all ages seek the help of their family doctor or dermatologist. Unfortunately, few, if any, conventional doctors ever relate the condition to nutrition or to vitamin D deficiency. Rather, the usual treatment involves a lifetime of corticosteroid creams and, in severe cases, oral cortisone prescriptions.

Fortunately, new research strongly suggests that long-term vitamin D supplementation would be very effective. Richard Gallo of the University of California has shown that taking vitamin D supplements boosts the production of a protective chemical substance that is normally present in the skin and which prevents skin infections as well as eczema. The more severe form of eczema, which is known as atopic dermatitis and affects approximately 10–20 percent of children, can be substantially improved or eliminated with adequate vitamin D supplements. Symptoms that can be improved include itching, redness, and scaling.

Skin infections like those caused by *Staphylococcus aureus* and herpes can also be prevented or curtailed by adequate supplementation with vitamin D. The main reason why vitamin D helps both eczema and skin infections is that it increases the production of a protein called cathelicidin, which has a protective effect against invading microbes and subsequent damage to the skin. The doses used in the study were 4,000 IU of vitamin D_3 for twenty-one days. The conclusion of the researchers follow: "These results suggest that supplementation with oral vitamin D dramatically induces cathelicidin production in the skin of patients with atopic dermatitis."

Epilepsy and Seizure Disorders

Research done recently at Boston University School of Medicine has revealed that almost half of all patients with epilepsy are vitamin D deficient. This is very important information because, prior to this study, the majority of epilepsy victims had no known cause of their seizure disorder. Remember that vitamin D receptors can be found in the brain, and these may well be important in balancing electrical activity in the brain. According to principal investigator Ionnis Karakis, "These results point out that vitamin D deficiency is very prevalent in the seizure population and that men are equally or even more often affected than women and therefore should not be overlooked or neglected."

It is also well known that antiepileptic medication can deplete vitamin D, folic acid, and other nutrients. Even those who do not have a conclusive vitamin D deficiency could eventually become dependent on vitamin D supplements if they haven been on long-term drug therapy.

Falls and Fractures in the Elderly

Falls among the elderly are a frequent occurrence, leading to significant morbidity and mortality. A 2006 study indicates that vitamin D deficiency is also related to the risk of falls and potential fractures in the elderly. The risk of falls can be reduced by increasing the blood levels of vitamin D. A supplement of 800 IU daily was found to cut the number of falls among elderly people in nursing homes by 70 percent.

Fertility

A recent infertility study has shown that vitamin D deficiency was an important factor in men who were unable to impregnate their partners. At least one-third of all men with fertility problems in this study had low blood levels of vitamin D.

Australian fertility specialist and study leader Anne Clark was quoted as saying, "Vitamin D and folate deficiency are known to be associated with infertility in women, but the outcomes of the screening among men in our study group came as a complete surprise. Men in the study group who agreed to make lifestyle changes and take dietary supplements had surprisingly good fertility outcomes."

Of course, there's much more to enhancing male fertility than just taking vitamin D. When most people think of enhancing male fertility, they think of boosting certain hormone levels. Testosterone, DHEA, growth hormone, estrogen, and progesterone are the major hormones involved, and their optimal levels in the body can be achieved without the use of prescription hormones in most people. It is now known that vitamin D blood levels are related to optimal levels of all the hormones involved with fertility.

To aid fertility, an optimal dose of vitamin D would be 10,000 IU daily if sunshine exposure has been lacking. To read more about male fertility, see my book *Boosting Male Libido Naturally* (Alive Books, 2000), available at naturals food stores.

Hearing Loss

If you are losing your hearing, get your blood levels of vitamin D checked. Studies now indicate that hearing loss can be prevented and even reversed by vitamin D supplementation. Vitamin D controls the amount of calcium that gets deposited or not deposited in the inner ear. If you have no access to a doctor, just make sure you get at least twenty minutes of direct sunlight exposure every day. If you cannot get access to sunshine, it's just as safe to supplement with at least 10,000 IU of vitamin D every day until your hearing returns to normal.

Inflammation

If you have inflammation (arthritis, iritis, pancreatitis, thyroiditis, or anything ending in "itis"), you need more vitamin D. One way that doctors measure the amount of inflammation present in the body is through a blood test called C-reactive protein (CRP). A modified version of this test, called high-sensitivity C-reactive protein (hs-CRP), is a good predictor for heart attack risk. The higher the number for CRP or hs-CRP, the more inflammation is present in the body. Researchers have demonstrated that if a person supplements with vitamin D, the CRP level goes down. For this reason, vitamin D can be said to be anti inflammatory.

In my private medical practice, I have been ordering hs-CRP, erythrocyte sedimentation rate (ESR), and fibrinogen blood tests for many years. Both ESR and fibrinogen are lab tests similar to the CRP test and indicate the levels of inflammation in the body. Once again, the higher the numbers with these tests, the higher the level of inflammation in the body. People suffering from active coronary artery disease, arthritis, autoimmune diseases like rheumatoid arthritis or lupus, cancer, infections, severe allergies, and skin rashes of any kind will often have one or more of these inflammation markers elevated.

Although I have never documented the fact as a published study, I have observed that the higher the lab values for these tests, the sicker the patient. In fact, critically ill patients generally have the lowest blood levels of vitamin D. Almost without exception, the higher the level of inflammation, the lower the blood level of vitamin D. Additionally, as vitamin D blood levels gradually increased in these patients via supplementation or greater sun exposure, the inflammatory markers decreased and the clinical outcomes for the patients improved.

The dosage of vitamin D needed to produce an anti-inflammatory effect may have to be much higher than 10,000 IU, so medical supervision would be required. Have your vitamin D blood levels checked and supplement accordingly if you cannot get enough sunshine.

If you have inflammation, you need more vitamin D. The dosage of vitamin D to produce an anti-inflammatory effect may have to be much higher than 10,000 IU, so medical supervision would be required.

Insomnia

There are many causes of insomnia or sleep disturbances of other types, but one of the most ignored may well be a deficiency in vitamin D. We now know that vitamin D is important for the proper functioning of the nervous system. We also know that conditions such as anxiety and depression are often associated with sleep disturbances and can be helped by increasing the blood levels of vitamin D.

If you suffer from sleep problems, ask your doctor to check your blood level of 25-hydroxy vitamin D. If it is below 200, vitamin D supplementation of 10,000 IU daily would certainly be worth a trial.

Kidney Disease

The August 2008 *Journal of the American Society of Nephrology* reports that treating patients who have moderate to severe chronic kidney disease with vitamin D reduces the risk of death by 25 percent. This is something that is normally accomplished with a prescription vitamin D analogue (calcitriol).

Chronic kidney disease may prevent the formation of active vitamin D, a process that usually occurs in the healthy kidney. If someone with chronic kidney disease develops a vitamin D deficiency, the risk of death from all causes naturally increases. Ensuring adequate blood levels of vitamin D in people suffering from chronic kidney disease may be life-saving.

Liver Disease

Research done at the University of Tennessee has found that 92.4 percent of patients who suffer from chronic liver disease (hepatitis or cirrhosis) are deficient in vitamin D. This should not be too surprising, since vitamin D metabolism involves the presence of healthy liver enzymes. According to lead researcher Nair Satheesh, "Since deficiency is common among these patients, vitamin D replacement may hopefully prevent osteoporosis and other bone complications related to end-stage liver disease."

Does vitamin D supplementation cause liver toxicity? Does it cause fatty liver? After all, fish and many other animals store vitamin D in the liver. The truth is that vitamin D deficiency can lead to liver failure and that using supplements to achieve normal vitamin D levels reverses liver disease. In people with nonalcoholic fatty liver disease (NAFLD), a growing problem in North America thought to be caused by insulin resistance, the levels of vitamin D are usually quite low, and liver dysfunction can be brought back to normal with adequate vitamin D supplementation. A 2007 study concludes that vitamin D_3 may play a role in reducing both the development and progression of NAFLD.

Lung Function

Respiratory researchers have found a strong correlation between the blood levels of vitamin D and a very sensitive lung-function test called FEV_1. The higher the vitamin D level, the better the lung function.

This finding has strong implications for anyone suffering from asthma, chronic bronchitis, emphysema, or pulmonary fibrosis. Greater sun exposure as well as supplementation with vitamin D is warranted. Blood tests for vitamin D and calcium levels should be done every three months to monitor progress. Vitamin D supplementation does not interfere with any medications prescribed for lung disease.

Macular Degeneration

As we age, the macula, an area at the back of the retina responsible for our sharpest vision, starts to degenerate, leading to the most common form of blindness among older adults in the United States. The condition has been termed age-related macular degeneration (AMD), and it affects over seven million people age forty and older in the United States. As our population ages, we can expect the incidence of this condition to increase over the next two decades.

Many nutrients are involved in reversing or at least improving the severity of AMD. According to recent research, vitamin D may play a crucial role in the prevention of early AMD. Researchers discussing their findings published in the *Journal of the American Medical Association* were quoted as saying, "Levels of serum vitamin D were inversely associated with early AMD but not advanced AMD."

To help those who suffer from AMD, a number of dietary changes can be made and a number of supplements can be taken. Here's what I usually recommend:

• Eat more legumes, which have a cleansing effect due to their high content of sulfur-containing amino acids.

• Eat more fresh fruits and vegetables, especially yellow vegetables. Berries are wonderful, particularly blueberries, because of their high content of anthocyanidins, and cherries because they offer carotenes, flavonoids, and vitamins C and E. Carotenoids, especially lutein and zeaxanthin, are most strongly associated with a reduced risk of macular degeneration. The best sources are collard greens, kale, and spinach.

In addition, take the antioxidant and eye-health-enhancing supplements shown in table 2 each day.

TABLE 2 DAILY SUPPLEMENTS FOR EYE HEALTH

Supplement	Dose
beta-carotene	100,000 IU
coenzyme Q10	100 mg, 3 times daily
high-carotenoid green drink, such as Bioquest brand Green Alive	1 tablespoon (15 mL) in water or juice
pycnogenol (from either pine bark extract or grape seed extract)	300 mg
selenium	600 mcg
vitamin C	2,000 mg, 3 times daily
vitamin D	10,000 IU
vitamin E	400 IU, 3 times daily
zinc chelate or citrate	100 mg

Research reveals that the following botanical medicines also show impressive results with this condition:

- bilberry (*Vaccinium myrtillus*), 80 mg twice daily, 25 percent anthocyanidin content
- ginkgo biloba extract, 250 mg

Bilberry is used in Europe for diabetic retinopathy cataracts, macular degeneration, and retinitis pigmentosa. Bilberry also prevents further damage from glaucoma by working as an antioxidant in the eyes. Its anthocyanidins increase intracellular vitamin C levels (vitamin C is a critical nutrient for healthy eyes) and decrease capillary fragility.

None of these natural supplements have any serious side effects. Regular blood tests every three months should be done to ensure your supplementation is at safe levels, and visits to the eye doctor to monitor your AMD are a good idea.

Migraines

According to research done in 2008, vitamin D deficiency is common in those suffering from chronic migraine headaches. This observation was first presented by Steve Wheeler of the Ryan Wheeler Headache Treatment Center in Miami at the 50th Annual Meeting of the American Headache Society. Wheeler reported that 41.8 percent of those who have chronic migraines were deficient in vitamin D. The longer a person suffers from migraines, the more likely the existence of vitamin D deficiency.

Wheeler, himself a migraine sufferer, was quoted as saying, "The first person I tested was myself, and I found I was severely vitamin D deficient (with a 25-hydroxy vitamin D level of 8.2 ng/ml). Levels greater than 30 ng/ml are considered sufficient, but only for bone health. Optimal levels for other conditions, such as cardiovascular disease, are still unknown, although it is believed they should be much higher."

He further went on to say, "Clinicians generally don't recognize the importance of vitamin D deficiency, and so they don't screen for it—not just in migraineurs, but in all of their patients. But it is a condition that is easily treated and may confer major, wide-ranging health benefits."

Vitamin D deficiency is common in those suffering from chronic migraine headaches.

Pain, Chronic Fatigue Syndrome, and Fibromyalgia

About ten years ago, a forty-five-year-old real estate agent came to see me because she had been suffering for the past five years from what had been diagnosed as fibromyalgia syndrome. She was suffering from generalized muscle and joint pain, chronic fatigue, insomnia, recurrent flulike illnesses, and poor cognitive function. Standard blood tests, X-rays, CAT scans, and other exotic tests failed to reveal any cause for her symptoms. She had been unable to work for the past year due to her health problems and had already seen at least a dozen doctors in a vain attempt to get some relief so she could return to work. None of them bothered to do a blood test for vitamin D. She had even seen a psychiatrist, who basically told her that she may be suffering from a form of depression and needed a six-month course of two different antidepressants. Some of the doctors she had consulted told her that she should not take any vitamins or minerals because they would be more likely to produce toxicity in someone as sick as she was.

This lady had been prescribed at least twenty-five different drugs that included a long list of analgesics, antidepressants, and tranquilizers. She arrived at my office in the hopes of finding some way to reverse her symptoms naturally. She was not a believer in natural therapies and was only consulting me on the strong urgings of one of her best friends.

After I received the results of her lab tests, I discovered that her blood level of 25-hydroxy vitamin D was extremely low at 10 ng/ml. This was a patient who was frightened to death of even minimal sun exposure and slathered on lots of sunscreen during the summer months when she ventured outdoors for any longer than twenty minutes. I prescribed 4,000 IU daily which, at the time, was considered to be an excessively high-dose prescription for vitamin D. Most doctors were prescribing close to 400 IU daily for osteoporosis and not even ordering blood tests for vitamin D. I prescribed vitamin D_3 in water-soluble drop form and told her to take four drops (4,000 IU) daily. Fortunately or unfortunately, she did not hear this advice correctly and took *forty* drops each day. She went for lab tests six weeks later and reported back to me at eight weeks. All of her symptoms were gone and she was ready to return to work. She had started to feel better at the three-week point, and her symptoms gradually disappeared over the next five weeks. Luckily, there were no side effects.

Her blood tests showed that her vitamin D levels had gone up two hundred points to 210 ng/ml and her ionized blood calcium level was within the normal range. Incidentally, I always check the blood calcium levels of

THE FALSE HOPE OF THE MARSHALL PROTOCOL

I have witnessed a lot of crazy treatments over the past thirty years, but none are as abusive as the Marshall protocol. This protocol is not only illogical but also downright dangerous. At best, it can be labeled as a pretense of scientific thought. I am including this information here because many people suffering from chronic fatigue syndrome, fibromyalgia, and other chronic health problems are using the protocol in the hopes of a cure. Many are so locked into the protocol that they refuse to hear how they may be damaging their health.

In brief, a few years ago an electrical engineer by the name of Trevor Marshall (who is not a doctor of anything except electrical engineering) formulated an elaborate opinion in a publication called *Science Daily*. This was neither a study nor anything scientific but was strictly based on the anecdotal experience of one individual who claims to have cured himself using the Marshall protocol.

What Marshall believes is that vitamin D originating from sunlight is different from that derived from oral supplements and is somehow toxic to the immune system. He also believes that the low levels of vitamin D found in many chronic diseases are the *result* of the disease and not its cause. Finally, his hypothesis is that taking any amount of vitamin D will make many of these inflammatory or autoimmune diseases worse, not better.

Marshall believes that the way to recover from chronic disease is to become very vitamin D deficient. This theory has never been proved by any scientific study or statistics. In fact, the opposite has been proved to be the case as evidenced by the very long list of studies referenced at the back of this book.

People who are treating themselves with the Marshall protocol wear wrap-around sunglasses to prevent any exposure whatsoever to sunlight. They wear large floppy hats and clothing that obstructs any sunlight contact with the skin. They are very careful to cover up any exposed skin that might accidentally come in contact with sunlight. Aside from this, patients are prescribed an angiotensin II receptor blocker and a variety of long-term antibiotics (for months or years), supposedly to repair the damage caused by vitamin D and to reactivate the immune system. The protocol is designed to be used for a period of three to five years.

For the sake of argument as well as to educate those who believe in the false hope provided by the Marshall protocol, let us examine the evidence more closely.

First, vitamin D behaves exactly the same in the body whether it is derived from sunlight or from an oral nutritional supplement. This is just basic science and has never been disproved by any study. Second, with respect to many diseases, especially those involving the nervous system, it has clearly been established that the lower the level of vitamin D, the worse the disease. For example, in the case of dementia, numerous studies have documented improved cognitive function in people who received vitamin D and whose blood levels increased. The lower the blood level of vitamin D, the worse the dementia. To say the opposite makes no sense whatsoever.

Sunlight exposure can cause dangerously high blood calcium levels in those afflicted with a disease known as sarcoidosis. Marshall suffered from this disease and claims to have cured himself by avoiding vitamin D and taking prescription antihypertensive drugs and antibiotics. In sarcoidosis, the body seems to lose its ability to regulate the production and proper utilization of vitamin D. This is the disease that Marshall uses as an example of how vitamin D from sunlight is toxic. The truth is that sarcoidosis is the only known disease in which vitamin D regulation in the body fails. No one really knows what causes this disease or why vitamin D regulation fails. To say it is caused by the mere presence of vitamin D is unproven.

According to adherents of the Marshall theory, the low levels of vitamin D seen in cancer are the *result of* as opposed to the *cause* of the cancer. This concept has resoundingly been refuted by the work of Creighton University researcher Joanne Lappe, who showed in a randomized controlled trial that baseline blood levels of vitamin D were strong and independent predictors of who would get cancer in the future. The lower the blood level of vitamin D, the greater the cancer risk.

The use of the Marshall protocol is damaging to one's health and can lead to death. I could not put it in any stronger terms. Marshall does not even have a biology degree. Although he labels himself "doctor," this is clearly a very loose use of the title. If one has a PhD in mathematics, one can technically be called "doctor." His title should therefore not in any way provide him with a measure of credibility. Marshall is an Australian electrical engineer. He may know electronics, but he certainly doesn't understand much about the human body. If you have been misled into using his protocol, do yourself a big favor and get off of it immediately.

patients who are using vitamin D supplements because vitamin D toxicity can cause dangerously high levels of calcium. Vitamin D toxicity was not the case in this patient despite the accidentally "toxic" supplementation levels. Now, before all you folks suffering from chronic pain start taking massive doses of vitamin D, please get your blood levels checked, and check them again after high-dose supplementation.

Insufficient amounts of vitamin D have been linked to a greater incidence of chronic fatigue, fibromyalgia syndrome, migraine headaches, muscle weakness, musculoskeletal pain, and numerous other conditions that cause pain. In the majority of cases involving pain, regardless of the cause of the pain, vitamin D supplementation will be helpful. The only question is at what dose. To find out, it's best to work with a qualified natural health care provider.

In the majority of cases involving pain, regardless of the cause of the pain, vitamin D supplementation will be helpful. The only question is at what dose.

Obesity

Vitamin D levels are significantly lower in overweight individuals, possibly because they have greater body mass that needs to be nourished compared to normal-weight individuals. Taking a vitamin D supplement may make all the difference in the world for people who are trying to lose weight.

Studies show that sunlight exposure and vitamin D levels somehow normalize food intake and blood sugar levels. If the body is deficient in vitamin D, the synthesis of fatty acids can increase as much as five times. The lower your blood level of vitamin D, the more your body manufactures fat and the heavier you get.

"Our results suggest the possibility that the addition of vitamin D to a reduced-calorie diet will lead to better weight loss," said Shalamar Sibley at the Endocrine Society's 91st Annual Meeting in Washington, DC, on June 12, 2009. In a 2008 study by scientists at McGill University and the University of Southern California, vitamin D deficiency was found to cause higher body mass and shorter stature in adolescent girls at the peak of their growing spurt.

When there is vitamin D deficiency, the body starts making more of an enzyme called fatty acid synthase by as much as fivefold. This enzyme converts calories into fat storage. Both higher calcium and vitamin D levels inhibit this enzyme. In other words, low blood levels of vitamin D mean more fat storage in the body.

The lower your blood level of vitamin D, the more your body manufactures fat and the heavier you get.

Osteoporosis

In North America, at least 30 percent of the population will get osteoporosis, a major cause of fractures and disability in the elderly adult population. Vitamin D plays a very important role in prevention, but this condition also is associated with a large number of other factors that must be considered.

While you can do nothing directly about your family history of osteoporosis, you can at least eliminate the majority of the following known risks of getting the disease:

- antacid abuse, antiulcer drugs
- anticoagulants (blood thinners)
- antiseizure medications
- cigarette smoking
- digestive disorders leading to trace-mineral malabsorption
- diuretics (water pills)
- drinking exclusively distilled water

- excessive alcohol and caffeine intake
- excessive physical exercise
- for women, never having been pregnant
- high consumption of milk and dairy products
- high sugar intake
- high-protein diets (animal protein encourages high mineral losses in the urine)
- inadequate exposure to sunlight or UVB light
- long-term use of prescription steroids like prednisone
- low-calorie weight-loss diets
- numerous vitamin and mineral deficiencies
- overactive endocrine glands (especially hyperthyroidism)
- physical inactivity

Regardless of what prescription or natural remedies you are using to fight osteoporosis, nothing can take the place of daily weight-bearing exercise. Unless the bones are challenged to function, no amount of calcium, estrogen, or any other remedy, for that matter, will make a difference in bone-mineral density. In other words, use it or lose it. Brisk walking, using arm and ankle weights, sit ups, leg lifts, and dozens of other exercises can be done with the help of a chiropractor, physiotherapist, or personal trainer.

As with all our body tissues, bone is sensitive to diet and lifestyle habits. The typical Western diet—which is high in refined carbohydrates, animal protein and fat, and canned and processed foods—has been linked to a greater incidence of osteoporosis simply because such a diet is inadequate in a large number of nutrients. It is also excessively high in phosphorus, a mineral that, in large amounts, reduces calcium in the body.

Interestingly enough, the foods most often recommended for healthy bones—milk and dairy products—are excessively high in phosphorus and may actually promote osteoporosis. In fact, people who consume the most dairy products have the worst osteoporosis incidence. In areas of the world where dairy product consumption is the lowest, osteoporosis is virtually nonexistent. Despite being fortified with vitamin D, milk fails to provide enough of the vitamin to prevent osteoporosis.

Since refined sugar contains virtually no vitamins or minerals at all, it dilutes our nutrient intake, resulting in an across-the-board 19 percent reduction in all vitamins and minerals in our diet. As a result, we are getting less copper, folic acid, magnesium, manganese, vitamin B_6, zinc, and other nutrients that play a role in maintaining healthy bones.

When whole wheat is refined to white flour, many vitamins and minerals are lost: calcium (60 percent), copper (68 percent), folic acid (67 percent), magnesium (85 percent), manganese (86 percent), vitamin B_6 (72 percent), and zinc (78 percent). Since grains make up about 30 percent of the average diet, consumption of refined grains depletes the total daily intake of micronutrients (vitamins and minerals).

Caffeine in analgesics, chocolate, coffee, herbs (such as guarana and yerba maté), and soft drinks cause the body to lose water and minerals, leading to lower bone mineral density. Similarly, excess alcohol causes abnormal mineral losses.

Excessive dietary protein (especially animal protein) may promote bone loss. With increasing protein intake, the urinary excretion of calcium also rises because calcium is mobilized to buffer the acidic breakdown products of protein. In addition, the amino acid methionine is converted to a substance called homocysteine, which is also capable of causing bone loss.

It continues to amaze me how many older adults suffer from conclusive vitamin D deficiency. I see it every day on blood test results and in the pale complexions of sun-phobic individuals. Vitamin D is required for us to absorb calcium from the small intestine. Deficiency can come about when there is reduced exposure to sunlight, decreased dietary intake, or a malabsorption problem of one kind or another. As we age, the ability to absorb all nutrients decreases and often necessitates the use of digestive enzyme capsules or other digestive aids. One way to overcome this is to use an emulsified form of vitamin D (a water-soluble form of a fat-soluble vitamin). Of course, regardless of what the dermatologists say, safely expose yourself as much as possible to sunlight and avoid sunscreens.

People who consume the most dairy products have the worst osteoporosis incidence. In areas of the world where dairy product consumption is the lowest, osteoporosis is virtually nonexistent.

Parkinson's Disease

Parkinson's disease involves the deterioration of specific nerve centers in the brain. This deterioration changes the chemical balance of acetylcholine and dopamine, two chemicals that are essential for transmitting nerve signals. When the balance between these two neurotransmitters is altered, the ultimate result is a lack of control of physical movements.

The five main symptoms and signs of Parkinson's disease are tremor, rigidity, bradykinesia (slowed movement), gait disorder, and loss of balance. Tremor is an involuntary shaking of the hands, the head, or both. Symptoms appear slowly, in no particular order, and some time may elapse before they interfere with normal activities. In many cases, this is accompanied by a continuous rubbing together of the thumb and forefinger. Stooped posture, a masklike face, trouble swallowing, depression, and difficulty performing simple tasks may all be seen at different stages of the disease. The tremors are most severe when the affected part of the body is not in use. There is no pain or other sensation other than a decreased ability to move. In severe cases, the person will be unable to walk smoothly due to an inability to swing the arms. Writing legibly and speaking clearly will also be affected.

Parkinson's disease affects more men than women at a ratio of three to two. It is estimated that one in every one hundred people over age sixty will contract this condition. Parkinson's occurs at the rate of 228 per 100,000 people and usually begins between the ages of fifty and sixty-five. It is much more prevalent in the age group of sixty to sixty-nine but is sometimes seen in patients under forty years of age, with an incidence of 10 per 100,000. The specific cause of Parkinson's disease is not known. Predisposing factors include carbon monoxide poisoning, high body levels of noxious chemicals, brain infections (encephalitis), and certain psychiatric drugs. Medical treatment involves the use of prescription drugs such as deprenyl, levodopa, and Sinemet (carbidopa-levodopa), all of which control symptoms for some years but eventually become ineffective. There is no medical cure for the condition, with all current treatments being primarily symptom suppressive, supportive, or palliative.

A 2008 study from Emory University School of Medicine showed that the majority of Parkinson's disease patients suffer from insufficient blood levels of vitamin D. It is now well established that degenerative brain disease can result from vitamin D deficiency. What is not known is whether giving vitamin D supplements to Parkinson's patients will make any difference in the course of their illness. Currently, a clinical trial at Emory University is under way to see whether supplementation of vitamin D in Parkinson's disease patients will be helpful. Certainly there could be a good case made for people who have Parkinson's disease in their family to supplement with vitamin D for prevention.

It is now well established that degenerative brain disease can result from vitamin D deficiency.

Psoriasis

The use of high-dose vitamin D supplementation for psoriasis has been known since 1986 to be an effective treatment. Most conventional doctors prescribe a vitamin D–analogue cream known as Dovonex (calcipotriene), with possibly a corticosteroid. According to Michael Holick, world expert on vitamin D therapy, "Among those who use Dovonex topically, upward of 50–60 percent have seen significant improvement." Megadose oral supplementation instead of or in addition to Dovonex use, will, unfortunately, not help in reversing psoriasis, a condition that is associated with many other nutritional factors beyond vitamin D.

Radiation Damage

Over the years, many people have asked me how they can prevent DNA and cell damage caused by different types of radiation. People are often concerned about X-rays and nuclear radiation from various medical investigations. Acute radiation damage can cause dehydration, nausea, skin reddening, or vomiting. Long-term exposure could increase the risk of cancer and birth defects. The answer to these concerns may well be vitamin D.

According to radiation expert Daniel Hays of the New York City Department of Health, "Our understanding and appreciation of the multi-protective actions of vitamin D have recently entered a new era. It is becoming recognized that its most active molecular form—1,25 dihydroxyvitamin D_3—may offer protection against a variety of radiation and otherwise induced damages. Its preventive/ameliorating actions should be given serious consideration as a protective agent against sublethal radiation injury and in particular that induced by low-level radiation."

Vitamin D regulates the cell cycle, and this involves growth, proliferation, differentiation, communication, programmed cell death (apoptosis), and the prevention of the formation of new blood vessels (antiangiogenesis).

Vitamin D allows for the production of certain proteins that help protect the cell and organs from damage caused by radiation.

Rickets and Osteomalacia

Rickets and osteomalacia are the same disease. In children the condition is called rickets, while the term "osteomalacia" is used for adults. In this disease, there is widespread bone pain and muscle weakness. In children, there is sometimes visible enlargement of the bones at joints, such as the wrists. Fractures can occur due to softening of the bones in general.

Even conventional medical practitioners who are completely unaware of the true value of vitamin D supplementation know this childhood bone disease is caused by extreme vitamin D deficiency. Rickets was the major reason why milk became fortified with tiny doses of the supplement. As we now know, however, the amount of vitamin D fortification in foods is inadequate.

Conventional doctors in the United States recommend what I consider to be a very small dose of 200 IU daily to prevent the disease, following the advice of the America Academy of Pediatrics. Combined with adequate sunshine exposure, this might be just enough to prevent the disease, but children who avoid sunshine and dairy products would do well to supplement at least 2,000 IU daily either in the form of cod liver oil or emulsified vitamin D drops such as Biotics Research Bio-D-Mulsion (see Resources, page 107).

Schizophrenia

Schizophrenia is a severely debilitating disease that affects at least one in one hundred adults in Canada. The condition is mostly controllable but incurable. People who suffer from this illness are likely to have a lifelong experience with it.

The good news is that Australian researchers have discovered that supplementing at least 2,000 IU of vitamin D in early life reduces the risk of schizophrenia in adult males. This makes sense because we know that there are vitamin D receptors in the brain, and optimal levels of vitamin D help normalize brain function and prevent conditions like autism, depression, and Parkinson's disease. Why not schizophrenia?

To quote the conclusion of these Australian researchers: "Vitamin D supplementation during the first year of life is associated with a reduced risk of schizophrenia in males. Preventing hypovitaminosis D during early life may reduce the incidence of schizophrenia." Further research needs to be done to see whether vitamin D supplementation can help improve or reverse the disease.

Australian researchers have discovered that supplementing at least 2,000 IU of vitamin D in early life reduces the risk of schizophrenia in adult males.

Septicemia

Septicemia is a life-threatening condition that occurs when bacteria invade the bloodstream. These bacteria release a poisonous substance called endotoxin, which causes most of the damage to the body during a bacterial invasion. The usual result of septicemia is multiple-organ failure and death. The condition is the cause of over five hundred thousand trips to the emergency room each year in the United States. In addition to this, at least 3 percent of all hospital admissions for all causes results in a case of sepsis. It is well known that patients who are admitted to hospitals have a much greater risk of acquiring an infection during their stay than if they were never admitted in the first place.

Interestingly enough, septicemia has its highest incidence during the winter months and its lowest in the fall. The rates of sepsis are also highest in northern latitudes and lowest in the southern latitudes. Deficiency of vitamin D plays a strong role because low levels of the vitamin prevent the production of cathelicidins, peptides that have a protective effect against invading microbes. The higher the level of vitamin D, the higher the cathelicidins and the lower the incidence of septicemia.

Tooth Decay

Inflamed gums? Recall that vitamin D is anti-inflammatory and has antibiotic properties. Cavities and gum disease are frequently associated with more serious, generalized illnesses such as Alzheimer's disease, dementia, diabetes, heart disease, respiratory infections, and other conditions. As many dentists will tell you, the state of the gums and teeth are well correlated with the general health of the individual. Recent research now shows strong evidence for vitamin D deficiency causing gum disease and cavities. Studies suggest that giving children high doses of vitamin D supplements prevents both problems.

Recent research now shows strong evidence for vitamin D deficiency causing gum disease and cavities.

Tuberculosis

It's been estimated that one-third of the world's population carries tuberculosis (TB) bacteria, but less than half a percent actually develops clinically significant disease. TB infects about nine million people a year and is spread by airborne bacteria that can settle in the lungs. Even though effective antibiotics are available, at least two million people die of TB each year.

Recent studies indicate that one of the major factors for determining whether an individual carrying TB develops an infection is vitamin D. In carriers, the greater the vitamin D deficiency, the more likely will be the development of a full-blown TB infection. In the 1800s and 1900s, long before we had expensive doctors and antibiotics, the successful treatment of TB was accomplished at sanatoriums, where TB victims were exposed to sunshine. This was also before the development of sunscreens. What this exposure did was increase blood levels of vitamin D.

The rise of AIDS and its adverse effects on immunity in the 1990s is thought to be partially responsible for the increased incidence of TB in the late twentieth century. Coupled with the increasing use of sunscreens, which further drive down the blood levels of vitamin D, it's easy to see why we have so many problems today with infectious disease, including TB.

If you have TB, the typical treatment involves the use of at least three different antibiotics for about a year. The good news is that one study showed a 100 percent cure of TB with a daily supplement of 10,000 IU of vitamin D. Vitamin D is postulated to work by increasing the production of a protein that kills the TB bacterium. If you happen to know anyone who has TB, get him or her into the sunshine and throw away those toxic sunscreens.

In the 1800s and 1900s, long before we had expensive doctors and antibiotics, the successful treatment of TB was accomplished at sanatoriums, where TB victims were exposed to sunshine.

5

Special Concerns for Women's Health

BACTERIAL VAGINAL INFECTIONS

The June 2009 issue of *The Journal of Nutrition* reports that vitamin D deficiency is associated with a higher incidence of bacterial vaginosis (BV), another term for bacterial vaginal infections. BV is associated with adverse pregnancy outcomes, and the higher the blood level of vitamin D, the lower the incidence of BV.

This finding should not be surprising given the strong antibiotic effect of vitamin D. The lower the vitamin D level, the higher the incidence of any infection.

C-SECTIONS

Caesarean sections involve a high-risk surgical procedure that could be avoided if the mother has adequate levels of vitamin D during pregnancy. Vitamin D deficiency may not be the only factor that leads to having a

C-section, but it is one of the preventable causes of unnecessary surgery. According to researchers who concluded a two-year study at Boston University School of Medicine in 2008, the lower the vitamin D blood levels, the higher the likelihood of the mother receiving a C-section.

In a medical news release, researcher Michael Holick was quoted as saying, "In our analysis, pregnant women who were vitamin D deficient at the time of delivery had almost four times the odds of a Caesarean birth than women who were not deficient." That means the chances of needing a C-section were four times greater.

Why is there such a great increase? Vitamin D deficiency can cause abnormalities in the brain, heart, and skeleton of the newborn as well as numerous biochemical imbalances that could cause anatomical and physiological abnormalities. Vitamin D deficiency also causes pelvic muscle and bone weakness, making it more difficult for the mother to deliver the baby vaginally.

PREECLAMPSIA

Preeclampsia is a potentially dangerous condition involving high blood pressure and protein in the urine of pregnant women. If left untreated, eclampsia can occur, resulting in maternal seizures and termination of the pregnancy. Although there may be other factors precipitating preeclampsia, such as a lack of protein, vitamin D deficiency has been discovered to be an independent risk factor for causing the condition.

Researchers have concluded that the known racial disparity in preeclampsia, with black women being more likely to develop severe preeclampsia and suffer greater morbidity associated with the disorder than white women, suggests vitamin D may be relevant. Moreover, the pathogenesis of preeclampsia involves a number of biological processes that may be directly or indirectly affected by vitamin D, including abnormal angiogenesis, excessive inflammation, hypertension, immune dysfunction, and placental implantation. If you happen to be pregnant, ask your doctor to check your 25-hydroxy vitamin D blood levels. It may make a huge difference in the outcome of your pregnancy.

PREMENSTRUAL SYNDROME (PMS)

Adequate blood levels of vitamin D reduce the risk of developing premenstrual syndrome (PMS), according to research published in the *Archives of Internal Medicine* in 2005. PMS symptoms may include abdominal bloating, fluid retention, headaches, irritability, and rapid mood swings.

Chief researcher, Elizabeth Bertone-Johnson, of the University of Massachusetts, stated, "We observed a significantly lower risk of developing PMS in women with high intakes of vitamin D and calcium from food sources, equivalent to about four servings per day of skim or low-fat milk, fortified orange juice, or low-fat dairy foods such as yogurt. These dietary intakes correspond to approximately 1,200 mg of calcium and 400 IU of vitamin D from food sources. While previous studies have observed the benefits of calcium supplements for treating PMS, this is the first, to our knowledge, to suggest that calcium and vitamin D may help prevent the initial development of PMS."

Of course, it goes without saying that some women will need higher doses of vitamin D than others. It all depends on the blood levels of 25-hydroxy vitamin D.

UTERINE FIBROIDS

About 30–70 percent of all women will have at least one fibroid in the uterus during their lifetime. Many of these women suffer from abdominal pain and abdominal bleeding leading to at least three hundred thousand hysterectomies in the United States every year.

Since vitamin D is an important modulator of many other hormones, it should not be surprising that uterine fibroids, a condition caused by an excess of estrogens relative to progesterone, can be reversed by optimizing vitamin D blood levels. African American women have as much as a 70 percent higher uterine fibroid rate than their white counterparts. Studies indicate that this is because levels of vitamin D generally are lower in black women.

Any woman suffering from uterine fibroids would certainly benefit from vitamin D supplementation. Blood levels, of course, would have to be tested on a regular basis to ensure safety.

References

Addy, R. 2009. "Harvard Backs Vitamin D Supplements." *NutraIngredients-usa.com.* Sept. 2. www.nutraingredients-usa.com/Industry/Harvard-backs-vitamin-D-supplements.

Aloia, J. F., and M. Li-Ng. 2007. "Re: Epidemic Influenza and Vitamin D." *Epidemiol Infect* 135 (7): 1095–96.

Anderson, P. G., C. H. Williams, H. Halderson, C. Summerfeldt, and R. Agnew. 1934. "Influence of Vitamin D in the Prevention of Dental Caries." *JADA* 21:1349–66.

Arnas, L. A. G., R. P. Heaney, and B. W. Hollis. 2004. "Vitamin D_2 Is Much Less Effective than Vitamin D_3 in Humans." Abstract OR22–2 presented at the Endocrine Society 86th Annual Meeting, New Orleans, LA.

Artaza, J. N., and K. C. Norris. 2009. "Vitamin D Reduces the Expression of Collagen and Key Profibrotic Factors by Inducing an Antifibrotic Phenotype in Mesenchymal Multipotent Cells." *J Endocrinol* 200:207–21.

Associated Content. 2008. "Can Vitamin D Prevent Skin Infections and Eczema?" Oct. 8. www.associatedcontent.com/article/1092194/can_vitamin_d_prevent_skin_infections.html?cat=5.

Baker, K., Y. Q. Zhang, and J. Goggins, et al. 2004. "Hypovitaminosis D and Its Association with Muscle Strength, Pain, and Physical Function in Knee Osteoarthritis." Abstract 1755 presented at the American College of Rheumatology Meeting, San Antonio, TX.

Barclay, L. 2009. "Vitamin D Deficiency Linked to Bacterial Vaginosis." *Medscape CME*, June 1. http://cme.medscape.com/viewarticle/703582?src=cmenews.

———. 2009. "Vitamin D Status Linked to Cognitive Function in Older Men." *Medscape CME*, June 2. http://cme.medscape.com/viewarticle/703659?src=cmenews.

Barclay, L., and P. Murata. 2007. "Maternal Vitamin D Deficiency May Increase the Risk for Preeclampsia." *Medscape CME*, June 6. http://cme.medscape.com/viewarticle/557673.

Bayer, R. 1960. "Treatment of Infertility with Vitamin E." *Int J Fertil* 5:70–78.

Beer, T. M., K. M. Eilers, M. Garzotto, M. J. Egorin, B. A. Lowe, and W. D. Henner. 2003. "Weekly High-Dose Calcitriol and Docetaxel in Metastic Androgen-Independent Prostate Cancer." *J Clin Oncol* 21:123–28.

Bertone-Johnson, E. R., et al. 2005. "Vitamin D and PMS." *Arch Intern Med* 165:1246–52.

Bhardwaj, A., A. Verma, S. Majumdar, and K. L. Khanduja. 2000. "Status of Vitamin E and Reduced Glutathione in Semen of Oligozoospermic and Azoospermic Patients." *Asian J Androl* 2 (3): 225–28.

Bhattoa, H. P., P. Bettembuk, S. Ganacharya, and A. Balogh. 2003. "Prevalence and Seasonal Variation of Hypovitaminosis D and Its Relationship to Bone Metabolism in Community-Dwelling Postmenopausal Hungarian Women." *Osteoporos Int*, Dec. 23.

Bischoff-Ferrari, H. A., M. Borchers, and F. Gudat, et al. 2004. "Vitamin D Receptor Expression in Human Muscle Tissue Decreases with Age." *J Bone Miner Res* 19:265–69.

Bjorn, L. O., and T. Wang. 2000. "Vitamin D in an Ecological Context." *Int J Circumpolar Health* 59:26–32.

Black, P. 2005. "Vitamin D and Pulmonary Function: A Survey: Discussion." *Medscape Today*. www.medscape.com/viewarticle/519358_4.

Brann, D. W., and V. B. Mahesh. 1997. "Excitatory Amino Acids: Evidence for a Role in the Control of Reproduction and Anterior Pituitary Hormone Secretion." *Endocr Rev* 18:678–700.

Brodsky, R. H., B. Schick, and H. Vollmer. 1941. "Prevention of Dental Caries by Massive Doses of Vitamin D." *Am J Dis Child* 62:1183–87.

Broe, K. E., T. C. Chen, J. Weinberg, H. A. Bischoff-Ferrari, M. F. Holick, and D. P. Kiel. 2007. "A Higher Dose of Vitamin D Reduces the Risk of Falls in Nursing Home Residents: A Randomized, Multiple-Dose Study." *J Am Geriatr Soc* 55 (October): 234–39.

Brookes, G. B. 1983. "Vitamin D Deficiency—A New Cause of Cochlear Deafness." *J Laryngol Otol* 97 (5): 405–20.

Canadian Cancer Society. 2007. "Canadian Cancer Society Announces Vitamin D Recommendation." June 8. www.cancer.ca/ccs/internet/mediareleaselist/ 0,3208,3172_1613121606_1997621989_langId-en,00.html (accessed June 13, 2007).

Cannell, J. J. 2003. "The Truth about Vitamin D Toxicity." *Vitamin D Council*. www.vitamindcouncil.org/vitaminDToxicity.shtml.

———. 2003. "Vitamin D and Mental Illness." *Vitamin D Council*. www.vitamindcouncil.org/mentalIllness.shtml.

———. 2008. "Cholecalciferol Is Cholecalciferol." *Vitamin D Council Newsletter*. April. www.vitamindcouncil.org/newsletter/2008-april.shtml.

Cannell, J. J., R. Vieth, J. C. Umhau, M. F. Holick, W. B. Grant, S. Madronich, C. F. Garland, and E. Giorvannucci. 2006. "Epidemic Influenza and Vitamin D." *Epidemiol Infect* 134:1129–40.

Cannell, J. J., M. Zasloff, C. F. Garland, R. Scragg, and E. Giovannucci. 2008. "On the Epidemiology of Influenza." *Virology J* 5:29. www.virologyj.com/content/5/1/29.

Cassels, C. 2007. "Vitamin D Deficiency Highly Prevalent Among Epilepsy Patients." *Medscape Today*, Dec. 6. www.medscape.com/viewarticle/567073.

———. 2008. "Vitamin D Deficiency Common in Patients with Chronic Migraine." *Medscape Today*, July 7. www.medscape.com/viewarticle/577151.

Chapuy, M. C., M. E. Arlot, and F. Duboeuf, et al. 1992. "Vitamin D_3 and Calcium to Prevent Hip Fractures in Elderly Women." *N Engl J Med* 327:1637–42.

Chiricone, D., N. G. De Santo, and M. Cirillo. 2003. "Unusual Cases of Chronic Intoxication by Vitamin D." *J Nephrol* 16:917–21.

Choi, Y. D., et al. 1997. "The Distribution of Nitric Oxide Synthase in Human Corpus Cavernosum on Various Impotent Patients." *Yonsei Med J* 38:125–132.

Costa, M., D. Canale, and M. Filicori, et al. 1994. "L-Carnitine in Idiopathic Asthenozoospermia: A Multicenter Study." *Andrologia* 26:155–59.

Crowle, A. J., E. J. Ross, and M. H. May. 1987. "Inhibition by 1,25(OH)2-Vitamin D_3 of the Multiplication of Virulent Tubercles Bacilli in Cultured Human Macrophages." *Infect Immun* 55 (12): 2945–50.

Cundy, T., S. A. Haining, D. F. Guilland-Cumming, J. Butler, and J. A. Kanis. 1987. "Remission of Hypoparathyroidism during Lactation: Evidence for a Physiological Role for Prolactin in the Regulation of Vitamin D Metabolism." *J Clin Endocrinol* 26 (6): 667–74.

Danai, P., et al. 2007. "Seasonal Variation in the Epidemiology of Sepsis." *Crit Care Med* 35:410–15.

Dawson, E. B., W. A. Harris, and L. C. Powell. 1990. "Relationship between Ascorbic Acid and Male Fertility." *World Rev Nutr Diet* 62:1–26.

Dawson-Hughes, B., S. S. Harris, E. A. Krall, and G. E. Dallal. 1997. "Effect of Calcium and Vitamin D Supplementation on Bone Density in Men and Women 65 Years of Age or Older." *N Engl J Med* 337:670–76.

Dawson-Hughes, B., R. P. Heaney, and M. F. Holick, et al. 2005. "Estimates of Optimal Vitamin D Status." *Osteoporos Int* 16:713–16.

De Aloysio, D., R. Mantuano, M. Mauloni, and G. Nicoletti. 1982. "The Clinical Use of Arginine Aspartate in Male Infertility." *Acta Eur Fertil* 13:133–67.

Deluca, H. F., and M. T. Cantorna. 2001. "Vitamin D: Its Role and Uses in Immunology." *FASEB J* 15:2579–85.

DeWinter, S., and S. Pavel. "Tanning Beds: Effect on Skin Cancer Risk Unclear." *Ned Tijdschr Geneeskd* 144 (10): 467–70.

Dhesi, J. K., C. Moniz, and J. C. Close, et al. 2002. "A Rationale for Vitamin D Prescribing in a Falls Clinic Population." *Age and Ageing* 31:267–71.

Di Cesar, D. J., R. Ploutz-Snyder, R. S. Weinstock, and A. M. Moses. 2006. "Vitamin D Deficiency Is More Common in Type 2 than in Type 1 Diabetes." *Diabetes Care* 29:174.

Dietrich, T., K. J. Joshipura, B. Dawson-Hughes, and H. A. Bischoff-Ferrari. 2004. "Association between Serum Concentrations of 25-Hydroxyvitamin D_3 and Periodontal Disease in the U.S. Population." *Am J Clin Nutr* 80:108–13.

Driver, J. P., O. Foreman, C. Mathieu., E. van Etten, and D. V. Serreze. 2008. "Comparative Therapeutic Effects of Orally Administered 1,25-Dihydroxyvitamin D_3 and 1Alpha-Hydroxyvitamin D_3 on Type-1 Diabetes in Non-Obese Diabetic Mice Fed a Normal Calcaemic Diet." *Clin Exp Immunol* 151 (1): 76–85.

Dye, C., S. Scheele, P. Dolin, V. Pathania, and M. C. Raviglione. 1999. "For the WHO Global Surveillance and Monitoring Project: Global Burden of Tuberculosis Estimated Incidence, Prevalence, and Mortality by Country." *JAMA* 282:677–86.

Embry, A. F. 2004. "Vitamin D Supplementation in the Fight against Multiple Sclerosis." *J Orthomolec Med* 19:27–38.

Environmental Working Group. 2009. Sunscreen Guide. www.ewg.org/whichsunscreensarebest/2009report.

Eureka Alert. 2008. "Vitamin D_2 Is as Effective as Vitamin D_3 in Maintaining Concentrations of 25-Hydroxyvitamin D." Jan. 2. www.eurekalert.org/pub_releases/2008-01/bu-vdi010208.php#.

Evatt, M. L., et al. 2008. "Prevalence of Vitamin D Insufficiency in Patients with Parkinson's Disease and Alzheimer's Disease." *Arch Neurol* 65:1348–52.

Eyles, D., J. Brown, A. Mackay-Sim, J. McGrath, and F. Feron. 2003. "Vitamin D_3 and Brain Development." *Neuroscience* 118:641–53.

Fallon, S., and M. G. Enig. 2004. "The Dangers of Statin Drugs: What You Haven't Been Told about Cholesterol-Lowering Medicines." *The Weston A. Price Foundation for Wise Traditions*, Spring 2004. www.westonaprice.org/moderndiseases/statin.html.

Flicker, L., K. Mead, and R. J. MacInnis, et al. 2003. "Serum Vitamin D and Falls in Older Women in Residential Care in Australia." *J Am Geriatr Soc* 51:1533–38.

Fuller, K., and J. M. Casparian. 2001. "Vitamin D: Balancing Cutaneous and Systemic Considerations." *Southern Med J* 94:58–66.

Gaby, A. 1994. *Preventing and Reversing Osteoporosis*. Rocklin, CA: Prima Publishing.

Garcion, E., N. Wion-Barbot, C. N. Montero-Menel, F. Berger, and D. Wion. 2002. "New Clues about Vitamin D Functions in the Nervous System." *Trends Endocrinol Metab* 13 (3): 100–05.

Ginde, A. A., J. M. Mansbach, and C. A. Camargo Jr. 2009. "Association between Serum 25-Hydroxyvitamin D Level and Upper Respiratory Tract Infection in the Third National Health and Nutrition Examination Survey." *Arch Intern Med* 169 (4): 384–90. http://archinte.ama-assn.org/cgi/content/abstract/169/4/384.

Glerup, H., K. Mikkelsen, and L. Poulsen, et al. 2000. "Commonly Recommended Daily Intake of Vitamin D Is Not Sufficient If Sunlight Exposure Is Limited." *J Intern Med* 247:260–68.

Godar, D. E., R. J. Landry, and A. D. Lucas. 2009. "Increased UVA Exposures and Decreased Cutaneous Vitamin D_3 Levels May Be Responsible for the Increasing Incidence of Melanoma." *Med Hypotheses* 72 (4): 434–43.

Goepp, J. 2009. "Vitamin D and Autism." *Life Extension Magazine*, April. www.lef.org/magazine/mag2009/apr2009_The-Link-Between-Autism-and-Low-Levels-of-Vitamin-D_01.htm.

Gonzales, G. F., et al. 2001."*Lepidium Meyenii* (Maca) Improved Semen Parameters in Adult Men." *Asian J Androl* 3 (4): 301–03.

Gorham, E. D., C. F. Garland, F. C. Garland, W. B. Grant, S. B. Mohr, M. Lipkin, H. L. Newmark, E. Giovannucci, M. Wei, and M. F. Holick. 2005. "Vitamin D and Prevention of Colorectal Cancer." *J Steroid Biochem Mol Biol* 97 (1–2): 179–94.

Gorham, E. D., et al. 2007. "Do Sunscreens Increase Risk of Melanoma in Populations Residing at Higher Latitudes?" *Ann Epidemiol* 17 (12): 956–63.

Goswami R., et al. 2009. "Prevalence of Vitamin D Deficiency and Its Relationship with Thyroid Autoimmunity in Asian Indians: A Community-Based Survey." *Br J Nutr* 10 (February): 1–5.

Grant, W. B. 2002. "An Ecologic Study of Dietary and Solar UVB Links to Breast Carcinoma Mortality Rates." *Cancer* 94:272–81.

———. 2002. "An Estimate of Premature Cancer Mortality in the United States Due to Inadequate Doses of Solar Ultraviolet-B Radiation." *Cancer* 94:1867–75.

———. 2004. "Geographic Variation of Prostate Cancer Mortality Rates in the United States: Implications for Prostate Cancer Risk Related to Vitamin D." *Int J Cancer* 111:470–71.

———. 2006. "How Strong Is the Evidence that Solar Ultraviolet B and Vitamin D Reduce the Risk of Cancer? An Examination Using Hill's Criteria for Causality." *Dermato Endocrinology* 1 (1): 4–6. www.landesbioscience.com/journals/dermatoendocrinology/article/Grant2DE1-1.pdf.

———. 2009. "Solar Ultraviolet-B Irradiance and Vitamin D May Reduce the Risk of Septicemia." *Dermato-Endocrinology* 1 (1): 1–6.

———. 2009. "A Critical Review of Vitamin D and Cancer: A Report of the IARC Working Group on Vitamin D." *Dermato-Endocrinology* 1 (1): 25–33.

———. 2009. "Does Vitamin D Reduce the Risk of Dementia?" *Alzheimers Dis* 17 (1): 151–9. www.j-alz.com/issues/17/vol17-1.html.

Grant, W. B., and C. F. Garland. 2006. "The Association of Solar Ultraviolet B (UVB) with Reducing Risk of Cancer: Multifactorial Ecologic Analysis of Geographic Variation in Age-Adjusted Cancer Mortality Rates." *Anticancer Res* 26:2687–99.

Grau, M. V., J. A. Baron, and R. S. Sandler, et al. 2003. "Vitamin D, Calcium Supplementation, and Colorectal Adenomas: Results of a Randomized Trial." *J Natl Cancer Inst* 95:1765–71.

Hanley, D., and K. S. Davison. 2005. "Symposium: Vitamin D Insufficiency: A Significant Risk Factor in Chronic Disease and Potential Disease-Specific Biomarkers of Vitamin D Sufficiency: Vitamin D Insufficiency in North America." *J Nutr* 135:332–37.

Hathcock, J. N., A. Shao, R. Vieth, and R. Heaney. 2007. "Risk Assessment for Vitamin D." *Am J Clin Nutr* 85:6–18.

Hayes, C. E. 2000. "Vitamin D: A Natural Inhibitor of Multiple Sclerosis." *Proceedings of the Nutrition Society* 59:531–535.

Hayes, D. P. 2008. "The Protection Offered by Vitamin D against Low Radiation Damage." *Int J Radiation* 5 (4): 368–94.

Herman, J. R., N. Krotkov, E. Celarier, E. Larko, and G. Labow. 1999. "Distribution of UV Radiation at the Earth's Surface from TOMS-Measured UV Backscattered Radiances." *J Geophys Res-Atmos* 104:12059–76.

Hidalgo, M., D. Rinaldi, G. Medina, T. Griffin, J. Turner, and D. D. Von Hoff. 1999. "A Phase I Trial of Topical Topitriol (Calcitriol, 1,25-Dihydoxyvitamin D_3) to Prevent Chemotherapy-Induced Alopecia." *Anticancer Drugs* 10 (4): 393–95.

Holick, M. F. 1987. "Photosynthesis of Vitamin D in the Skin: Effect of Environmental and Lifestyle Variables." *Fed Proc* 46:1876–82.

———. 1992. "Evolutionary Biology and Pathology of Vitamin D." *J Nutr Sci Vitaminol* (Tokyo), Spec No:79–83.

———. 2001. "Sunlight 'D'ilemma: Risk of Skin Cancer or Bone Disease and Muscle Weakness." *Lancet* 357:4–6.

———. 2003. "Vitamin D Deficiency: What a Pain It Is." *Mayo Clin Proc* 78 (12): 1457–59.

———. 2004. "Vitamin D: Importance in the Prevention of Cancers, Type 1 Diabetes, Heart Disease, and Osteoporosis." *Am J Clin Nutr* 79:362–71.

———. 2006. "Resurrection of Vitamin D Deficiency and Rickets." *J Clin Invest* 116 (8): 2062–72.

———. 2007. "Article Review: Vitamin D Deficiency." *NEJM Medical Progress* 357:266–81. www.uvadvantage.org/portals/0/pdf/NEJournalofMedicine.pdf.

——— 2009. "Shining Light on the Vitamin D–Cancer Connection IARC Report." *Dermato-Endocrinology* 1 (1): 4–6.

Holick, M. F., R. M. Biancuzzo, T. C. Chen, E. K. Klein, A. Young, D. Bibuld, R. Reitz, W. Salameh, A. Ameri, and A. D. Tannenbaum. 2007. "Vitamin D_2 Is as Effective as Vitamin D_3 in Maintaining Circulating Concentrations of 25-Hydroxyvitamin D." *J Clin Endocrinol Metab* 93:677–81.

Hollis, B.W. 2005. "Circulating 25-Hydroxyvitamin D Levels Indicative of Vitamin D Sufficiency: Implications for Establishing a New Effective Dietary Intake Recommendation for Vitamin D." *J Nutr* 135:317–22.

Hong, C. Y., B. N. Chiang, and P. Turner. 1984. "Calcium Ion Is the Key Regulator of Human Sperm Function." *Lancet* 2:1449–51.

Houghton, L., and R. Vieth. 2006. "The Case against Ergocalciferol (Vitamin D_2) as a Vitamin Supplement." *Am J Clin Nutr* 84:694–97.

Howard, J. E., and R. J. Meyer. 1948. "Intoxication with Vitamin D." *J Clin Endocrinol Metab* 8 (11): 895–910.

Huisman, A. M., K. P. White, and A. Algra, et al. 2001. "Vitamin D Levels in Women with Systemic Lupus Erythematosus and Fibromyalgia." *J Rheumatol* 28:2535–39.

Hunt, C. D., P. E. Johnson, J. Herbel, and L. K. Mullen. 1992. "Effects of Dietary Zinc Depletion on Seminal Volume and Zinc Loss, Serum Testosterone Concentrations, and Sperm Morphology in Young Men." *Am J Clin Nutr* 56:148–57.

Hypponen, E., E. Laara, A. Reunanen, M. R. Jarvelin, and S. M. Virtanen. 2001. "Intake of Vitamin D and Risk of Type 1 Diabetes: A Birth-Cohort Study." *Lancet* 358:1500–03.

Ingraham, B. A., B. Bragdon, and A. Nohe. 2008. "Molecular Basis of the Potential of Vitamin D to Prevent Cancer." *Curr Med Res Opin* 24:139–49.

The International Network of Cholesterol Skeptics Website. www.thincs.org.

Jablonski, N. G., G. Chaplin. 2000. "The Evolution of Human Skin Coloration." *J Hum Evol* 39:57–106.

Johansson, S., and H. Melhus. 2001. "Vitamin A Antagonizes Calcium Response to Vitamin D in Man." *J Bone Miner Res* 16:1899–905.

John, E. M., G. G. Schwartz, and J. Koo, et al. 2005. "Sun Exposure, Vitamin D Receptor Gene Polymorphisms, and Risk of Advanced Prostate Cancer." *Cancer Res* 65:5470–79.

Jorde, R., M. Sneve, Y. Figenschau, J. Svartberg, and K. Waterloo. 2008. "Effects of Vitamin D Supplementation on Symptoms of Depression in Overweight and Obese Subjects: Randomized Double Blind Trial." *J Intern Med* 264:599–609.

Karatekin, G., A. Kaya, O. Saltho lu, H. Balci, and A. Nuho lu. 2009. "Association of Subclinical Vitamin D Deficiency in Newborns with Acute Lower Respiratory Infection and Their Mothers." *Eur J Clin Nutr* 63 (4): 473–77.

Kenny, A. M., B. Biskup, and B. Robbins, et al. 2003. "Effects of Vitamin D Supplementation on Strength, Physical Function, and Health Perception in Older, Community-Dwelling Men." *J Am Geriatr Soc* 51:1762–67.

Khazai, N. B., S. E. Judd, L. Jeng, L. L. Wolfenden, A. Stecenko, T. R. Ziegler, and V. Tangpricha. 2009. "Treatment and Prevention of Vitamin D Insufficiency in Cystic Fibrosis Patients: Comparative Efficacy of Ergocalciferol, Cholecalciferol, and UV Light." *J Clin Endocrinol Metab* 94 (6): 2037–43.

Kimball, S. M., M. R. Ursell, P. O'Connor, and R. Vieth. 2007. "Safety of Vitamin D_3 in Adults with Multiple Sclerosis." *Am J Clin Nutr* 86:645–51.

Krall, E. A., C. Wehler, and R. I. Garcia, et al. 2001. "Calcium and Vitamin D Supplements Reduce Tooth Loss in the Elderly." *Am J Med* 111:452–56.

Kremer, R., et al. 2008. "Vitamin D Status and Its Relationship to Body Fat, Final Height, and Peak Bone Mass in Young Women." *J Clin Endocrinol Metab* 94:67–73.

Laaksi, I., J. P. Ruohola, P. Tuohimaa, A. Auvinen, R. Haataja, H. Pihlajamäki, and T. Ylikomi. 2007. "An Association of Serum Vitamin D Concentrations < 40 nmol/L with Acute Respiratory Tract Infection in Young Finnish Men." *Am J Clin Nutr* 86 (3): 714–17.

Lappe, J. M., D. Travers-Gustafson, K. M. Davies, R. R. Recker, and R. P. Heaney. 2007. "Vitamin D and Calcium Supplementation Reduces Cancer Risk: Results of a Randomized Trial." *Am J Clin Nutr* 85:1586–91.

Lin, J., J. E. Manson, and I. M. Lee, et al. 2007. "Intakes of Calcium and Vitamin D and Breast Cancer Risk in Women." *Arch Intern Med* 167:1050–59.

Lindeman, R. D. 1986. "Chronic Renal Failure and Magnesium Metabolism." *Magnesium* 5 (5–6): 300.

Liu, P. T., et al. 2006. "Toll-Like Receptor Triggering of a Vitamin D-Mediated Human Antimicrobial Response." *Science* 311:1770–73.

Liu, S., Y. Song, and E. S. Ford, et al. 2005. "Dietary Calcium, Vitamin D, and the Prevalence of Metabolic Syndrome in Middle-Aged and Older U.S. Women." *Diabetes Care* 28:2926–32.

London, M. 2008. "Is the Treatment for Sarcoidosis Helpful for Other Chronic Diseases? MP's Theories Are Not Supported by Lab Studies." *MIT Student Portal*. July 2. http://stuff.mit.edu/people/london/universe.htm.

McGrath, J., et al. 2004. "Vitamin D Supplementation during the First Year of Life and Risk of Schizophrenia: A Finnish Birth-Cohort Study." *Schizophrenia Research* 67:237–45.

Marshall Protocol Study Site. www.marshallprotocol.com.

Martins, D., M. Wolf, and D. Pan, et al. 2007. "Prevalence of Cardiovascular Risk Factors and the Serum Levels of 25-Hydroxyvitamin D in the United States." *Arch Intern Med* 167:1159–65.

Matsuoka, L. Y., J. Wortsman, N. Hanifan, and M. F. Holick. 1988. "Chronic Sunscreen Use Decreases Circulating Concentrations of 25-Hydroxyvitamin D: A Preliminary Study." *Arch Dermatol* 124:1802–04.

Maynard, M. T. 1938. "Vitamin D in Acne: A Comparison with X-Ray Treatment." *Cal West Med* 49 (2): 127–32.

McClean, T. 2008. "Lack of Sunlight Linked to Male Infertility." *News.com.au*, Oct. 19. www.news.com.au/story/0,23599,24519427-36398,00.html?from=public_rss.

Medical News Today. 2005. "Vitamin D Repletion Regimen for Cystic Fibrosis Patients Did Not Work." July 15. www.medicalnewstoday.com/articles/27487.php.

Medical News Today. 2008. "Vitamin D Linked to Reduced Mortality in Chronic Kidney Disease." May 9. www.medicalnewstoday.com/articles/106689.php.

Medical News Today. 2009. "Millions of U.S. Children Deficient in Vitamin D." Aug. 4. www.medicalnewstoday.com/articles/159668.php.

The Medical Post. 2009. "Vitamin D May Play a Role in Weight Loss Success." www.medicalpost.com/therapeutics/nutrition/article.jsp?content=20090721_101723_5792.

Melamed, M. L., E. D. Michos, W. Post, and B. Astor. 2008. "25-Hydroxyvitamin D Levels and the Risk of Mortality in the General Population." *Arch Intern Med* 168:1629–37.

Mercola.com. 2008. "Vitamin D Is a Key Player in Your Overall Health." Nov. 1. http://articles.mercola.com/sites/articles/archive/2008/11/01/Vitamin-D-is-a-Key-Player-in-Your-Overall-Health.aspx.

Merlino, L. A., J. Curtis, and T. R. Mikuls, et al. 2004. "Vitamin D Intake Is Inversely Associated with Rheumatoid Arthritis: Results from the Iowa Women's Health Study." *Arthritis Rheum* 50:72–77.

Minne, H. W., M. Pfeifer, and B. Begerow, et al. 2000. "Vitamin D and Calcium Supplementation Reduces Falls in Elderly Women Via Improvement of Body Sway and Normalization of Blood Pressure: A Prospective, Randomized, and Double-Blind Study." Abstract presented at the World Congress on Osteoporosis, Chicago, IL.

Mittelstaedt, M. 2007. "Sweeping Cancer Edict: Take Vitamin D Daily: Recommendation Comes on Heels of U.S. Study Suggesting Supplement Slashes Risk of Disease by as Much as 60 Percent." *Toronto Globe and Mail*, June 8.

Moncada, M. L., E. Vicari, and C. Cimino, et al. 1992. "Effect of Acetylcarnitine Treatment in Oligoasthenospermic Patients." *Acta Europaea Fertilitatis* 23:221–24.

MotherNature.com. "Prescription Vitamin D Delivers Hope for Psoriasis." www.mothernature.com/Library/Bookshelf/Books/10/98.cfm.

Mortia, R., I. Yamamoto, M. Takada, Y. Ohnaka, and I. Yuu. 1993. "Hypervitaminosis D." *Nippon Rinsho* 51 (4): 984–88.

Mouridsen, S. E., S. Nielsen, B. Rich, and T. Isager. 1994. "Season of Birth in Infantile Autism and Other Types of Childhood Psychoses." *Child Psychiatry Hum Dev* 25:31–43.

Muller, K., N. J. Kriegbaum, B. Baslund, O. H. Sorensen, M. Thyman, and K. Bentzen. 1995. "Vitamin D_3 Metabolism in Patients with Rheumatic Diseases: Low Serum Levels of 25-Hydroxyvitamin D_3 in Patients with Systemic Lupus Erythematosus." *Clin Rheumatol* 14:397–400.

Multiple Sclerosis Society of Canada. 2008. "World Congress on MS Takes Place in Montreal." *MSSociety.ca*, Oct. 2. www.mssociety.ca/en/research/medmmo_20081002.htm.

Munger, K. L., S. M. Zhang, and E. O'Reilly, et al. 2004. "Vitamin D Intake and Incidence of Multiple Sclerosis." *Neurology* 62:60–65.

Munger, K. L., L. I. Levin, B. W. Hollis, N. S. Howard, and A. Ascheino. 2006. "Serum 25-Hydroxyvitamin D Levels and Risk of Multiple Sclerosis." *JAMA* 296:2832–38.

NASA: Total Ozone Mapping Spectrometer. "DNA Spectral Exposure for July 1992" (compares skin cancer type and frequency by latitude). http://toms.gsfc.nasa.gov/ery_uv/dna_exp.gif (accessed Feb. 25, 2004).

National Institutes of Health. "Dietary Supplements Fact Sheet: Vitamin D." http://ods.od.nih.gov/factsheets/vitamind.asp.

Nesby-O'Dell S., K. S. Scanlon, and M. E. Cogswell, et al. 2002. "Hypovitaminosis D Prevalence and Determinants among African-American and White Women of Reproductive Age: Third National Health and Nutrition Examination Survey, 1988–1994." *Am J Clin Nutr* 76:187–92.

Netter, A., R. Hartoma, and K. Nahoul. 1981. "Effect of Zinc Administration on Plasma Testosterone, Dihydrotestosterone, and Sperm Count." *Arch Androl* 7:69–73.

Nursyam, E. W., Z. Amin, and C. M. Rumende. 2006. "The Effect of Vitamin D as Supplementary Treatment in Patients with Moderately Advanced Pulmonary Tuberculous Lesion." *Acta Med Indones* 38 (1): 3–5.

Oliva, A., et al. 2001. "Contribution of Environmental Factors to the Risk of Male Infertility." *Human Reproduction* 16:1768–76.

Omenn, G. S. 1996. "Micronutrients (Vitamins and Minerals) as Cancer-Preventive Agents." *IARC Sci Publ* 139:33–45.

Pain Treatment Topics. 2008. "Vitamin D—A Neglected 'Analgesic' for Chronic Musculoskeletal Pain." June. http://pain-topics.org/pdf/vitamind-briefing.pdf.

Pakkala, S., S. deVos. E. Elstner, R. K. Rude, M. Uskokovic, L. Binderup, and H. P. Koeffler. 1995. "Vitamin D_3 Analogs: Effect on Leukemic Clonal Growth and Differentiation, and on Serum Calcium Levels." *Leuk Res* 19:65–72.

Parekh, N. 2007. "Association between Vitamin D and Age-Related Macular Degeneration in the Third National Health and Nutrition Examination Survey 1988 through 1994." *Arch Ophthalmol* 125:661–69.

Piacentino, R., D. Malara, and F. Zaccheo, et al. 1991. "Preliminary Study of the Use of S. Adenosyl Methionine in the Management of Male Sterility" [in Italian]. *Minerva Ginecologica* 43:191–93.

Piazza, L., G. Liardo, A. DeMaria, L. Troiano, A. Terminella, and M. A. Cannizzaro. 1990. "Hypocalcemia after Total Thyroidectomy: Therapeutic Considerations." *Minerva Chir* 45 (18): 1161–63.

Pittas, A. G., B. Dawson-Hughes, and T. Li, et al. 2006. "Vitamin D and Calcium Intake in Relation to Type 2 Diabetes in Women." *Diabetes Care* 29:650–56.

Plotnikoff, G. A., and J. M. Quigley. 2003. "Prevalence of Severe Hypovitaminosis D in Patients with Persistent, Nonspecific Musculoskeletal Pain." *Mayo Clin Proc* 78:1463–70.

Pols, H. A. P., J. C. Birkenhauger, J. A. Foekens, and J. P. T. M. van Leeuwen. 1990. "Vitamin D: A Modulator of Cell Proliferation and Differentiation." *J Steroid Biochem Mol Biol* 37 (6): 873–76.

Ponsonby, A., A. McMichael, and I. van der Mei. 2002. "Ultraviolet Radiation and Autoimmune Disease: Insights from Epidemiological Research." *Toxicology* 181–182:71–78.

Preidt, R. 2008. "Vitamin D Deficit in Pregnancy Tied to Caesarean Risk." *HealthDay*. www.healthday.com/Article.asp?AID=622478.

Raloff, J. 2006. "The Antibiotic Vitamin: Deficiency in Vitamin D May Predispose People to Infection." *Science News*, Nov. 11. http://findarticles.com/p/articles/mi_m1200/is_20_170/ai_n16865477.

Richardson, A. 2009. "Vitamin D Impairs Low Level Radiation." *Suite101.com*. March 22. http://nutrition.suite101.com/article.cfm/vitamin_d_impairs_low_level_radiation#ixzz0Njgm9mRn.

Robsahm, T. E., S. Tretli, A. Dahlback, and J. Moan. 2004. "Vitamin D_3 from Sunlight May Improve the Prognosis of Breast, Colon, and Prostate Cancer (Norway)." *Cancer Causes & Control* 15:149–58.

Rona, Z. P. 1991. *Fertility Control—The Natural Approach*. Toronto: S. R. Vitamins.

Rona, Z. P., ed. 1998. *The Encyclopedia of Natural Healing*. Burnaby, BC: Alive Books.

Rona, Z. P. 2000. *Boosting Male Libido Naturally*. Vancouver: Alive Books.

Rosedale, R. "Cholesterol Is Not the Cause of Heart Disease." *DrRosedale.com*. www.drrosedale.com/resources/pdf/Cholesterol%20is%20NOT%20the%20cause%20of%20heart%20disease.pdf.

Salvati, G., G. Genovesi, and L. Marcellini, et al. 1996. "Effects of Panax Ginseng C.A. Meyer Saponins on Male Fertility." *Panmineva Med* 38:249–54.

Sandler, B., and B. Faragher. 1984. "Treatment of Oligospermia with Vitamin B_{12}." *Infertil* 7:133–38.

Sardi, B. 2007. "Just One Pill Away." *LewRockwell.com*. Feb. 20. www.lewrockwell.com/sardi/sardi70.html.

Schacter, A., J. A. Goldman, and Z. Zukerman. 1973. "Treatment of Oligospermia with the Amino Acid Arginine." *J Urol* 110:311–13.

Schleithoff, S., A. Zittermann, G. Tenderich, H. K. Berthold, P. Stehle, and R. Koerfer. 2006. "Vitamin D Supplementation Improves Cytokine Profiles in Patients with Congestive Heart Failure: A Double-Blind, Randomized, Placebo-Controlled Trial." *Am Journal Clin Nutr* 83:754–59.

Science Daily. 2008. "Vitamin D Deficiency Common in Patients with IBD, Chronic Liver Disease." Oct. 13. www.sciencedaily.com/releases/2008/10/081006092645.htm.

Science Daily. 2008. "Lack of Vitamin D Causes Weight Gain and Stunts Growth in Girls." Dec. 11. www.sciencedaily.com/releases/2008/12/081210122238.htm.

Secular Apostasy. 2008. "Vitamin D, Black American Women, and Fibroids." May 18. http://torduange.wordpress.com/2008/05/18/vitamin-d-black-american-women-and-fibroids.

Shah, M., N. Salhab, and D. Patterson, et al. 2000. "Nutritional Rickets Still Afflict Children in North Texas." *Tex Med* 96:64–68.

Shany, S., L. Yfat, and M. Lahav-Cohen. 2001. "The Effects of 1a,24(S)-Dihydroxyvitamin D_2 Analog on Cancer Cell Proliferation and Cytokine Expression." *Steroids* 66:319–23.

Shiizaki, K., I. Hatamura, S. Negi, T. Sakaguchi, F. Saji, I. Imazeki, E. Kusano, T. Shigematsu, and T. Akizawa. 2008. "Highly Concentrated Calcitriol and Its Analogues Induce Apoptosis of Parathyroid Cells and Regression of the Hyperplastic Gland—Study in Rats." *Nephrol Dial Transplant* 23 (5): 1529–36.

Sinatra, S. 2009. "Clearing Up the Cholesterol Confusion." *Townsend Letter*, June. www.townsendletter.com/June2009/clearingcholesterol0609.htm.

Steddon, S. J., N. J. Schroeder, and J. Cunningham. 2001. "Vitamin D Analogues: How Do They Differ and What Is Their Clinical Role?" *Nephrol Dial Transplant* 16:1965–67. http://ndt.oxfordjournals.org/cgi/content/full/16/10/1965.

Tangpricha, V., E. N. Pearce, T. C. Chen, and M. F. Holick. 2002. "Vitamin D Insufficiency Among Free-Living Healthy Young Adults." *Am J Med* 112 (8): 659–62.

Tangpricha, V., P. Koutkia, S. M. Rieke, T. C. Chen, A. A. Perez, and M. F. Holick. 2003. "Fortification of Orange Juice with Vitamin D: A Novel Approach for Enhancing Vitamin D Nutritional Health." *Am J Clin Nutr* 77:1478–83.

Targher, G., et al. 2007. "Associations between Serum 25-Hydroxyvitamin D_3 Concentrations and Liver Histology in Patients with Non-Alcoholic Fatty Liver Disease." *Nutr Metab Cardiovasc Dis* 17 (7): 517–24.

Termorshuizen, F., A. Wijga, J. Gerritsen, H. J. Neijens, and H. van Loveren. 2004. "Exposure to Solar Ultraviolet Radiation and Respiratory Tract Symptoms in One-Year-Old Children." *Photodermatol Photoimmunol Photomed* 20 (5): 270–71.

Terry, P., J. A. Baron, and L. Bergkvist, et al. 2002. "Dietary Calcium and Vitamin D Intake and Risk of Colorectal Cancer: A Prospective Cohort Study in Women." *Nutr Cancer* 43:39–46.

Trang, H. M., D. E. Cole, and L. A. Rubin, et al. 1998. "Evidence that Vitamin D_3 Increases Serum 25-Hydroxyvitamin D More Efficiently than Does Vitamin D_2." *Am J Clin Nutr* 68:854–58.

Tuohimaa, P., L. Tenkanen, and M. Ahonen, et al. 2004. "Both High and Low Levels of Blood Vitamin D Are Associated with a Higher Prostate Cancer Risk: A Longitudinal, Nested Case-Control Study in the Nordic Countries." *Int J Cancer* 108:104–08.

Turner, M. K., W. M. Hooten, J. E. Schmidt, J. L. Kerkvliet, C. O. Townsend, and B. K. Bruce. 2008. "Prevalence and Clinical Correlates of Vitamin D Inadequacy among Patients with Chronic Pain." *Pain Med*, March 11.

USDoctor.com. "Insomnia Information." www.usdoctor.com/insomnia.htm.

van Leeuwen J. P. T. M., and H. A. P. Pols. 2005. "Vitamin D: Cancer and Differentiation." In *Vitamin D*, eds. D. Feldman, F. H. Glorieux, J. W. Pike, 1571–97. San Diego: Elsevier Academic Press.

Vieth, R. 1999. "Vitamin D Supplementation, 25-Hydroxyvitamin D Concentrations, and Safety." *Am J Clin Nutr* 69:842–56.

Vitali, G., R. Parente, and C. Melotti. 1995. "Carnitine Supplementation in Human Idiopathic Asthenospermia: Clinical Results." *Drugs Exptl Clin Res* 21:157–59.

Wayse, V., A. Yousafzai, K. Mogale, and S. Filteau. 2004. "Association of Subclinical Vitamin D Deficiency with Severe Acute Lower Respiratory Infection in Indian Children Under Five." *Eur J Clin Nutr* 58 (4): 563–67.

Webb, A. R., and M. F. Holick. 1988. "Influence of Season and Latitude on the Cutaneous Synthesis of Vitamin D_3: Exposure to Winter Sunlight in Boston and Edmonton Will Not Promote Vitamin D_3 Synthesis in Human Skin." *J Clin Endocrinol Metab* 67 (2): 273-38.

Welsh, J. 2006. "Calcium and Vitamin D." In *Nutritional Oncology*, eds. G. Blackburn, V. Go, D. Heber, and J. Milner, 545–58. Burlington, MA: Elsevier Academic Press.

Wietrzyk, J., M. Petczynska, J. Madej, S. Dzimira, H. Kusnierczyk, A. Kutner, W. Szelejewski, and A. Opolski. 2004. "Toxicity and Antineoplastic Effect of (24R)-1-,24-Dihydroxyvitamin D_3 (PRI-2191)." *Steroids* 69 (10): 629–35.

Wolf, P., et al. 1998. "Phenotypic Markers, Sunlight-Related Factors, and Sunscreen Use in Patients with Cutaneous Melanoma: An Austrian Case-Control Study." *Melanoma Res* 8 (4): 370 78.

Woo, T. C., R. Choo, M. Jamieson, S. Chander, and R. Vieth. 2005. "Pilot Study: Potential Role of Vitamin D (Cholecalciferol) in Patients with PSA Relapse after Definitive Therapy." *Nutr Cancer* 51 (1): 32–36.

Zehnder, D., Y. C. Lin, H. Yang, M. Hewison, and J. S. Adams. 2004. "Measurement of Vitamin D Levels in Inflammatory Bowel Disease Patients Reveals a Subset of Crohn's Patients with Elevated 1,25-D and Low Bone Mineral Density." *Gut* 53 (8): 1129–36. www.ncbi.nlm.nih.gov/pubmed/15247180.

Zella, J. B., and H. F. DeLuca. 2003. "Vitamin D and Autoimmune Diabetes." *J Cell Biochem* 88:216–22.

Zouboulis, C. C. 2000. "Human Skin: An Independent Peripheral Endocrine Organ." *Horm Res* 54:230–42.

Resources

INFORMATION

Joseph Mercola
www.mercola.com
From his Natural Health Center in Illinois, Joseph Mercola publishes an online source of health articles, including one about more than thirty ailments that are helped by vitamin D.

Joe Prendergast
www.endocrinemetabolic.com
www.uncommondoctor.com
An endocrinologist and diabetologist, and the author of *Dr. Joe's Rx for Managing Your Health*, Joe Prendergast helps patients with diabetes, compromised immune systems, and heart disease modify their lifestyles and become less prone to distress and disease.

Norm Shealy
www.normshealy.com
One of the world's leading experts in pain management, Norm Shealy advocates "self-health" and is the founder of the American Holistic Medical Association and author of twenty-three books.

Vitamin D Council
www.vitamindcouncil.org
The Vitamin D Council website, managed by John Cannell, executive director, provides information about vitamin D deficiency and how it contributes to conditions such as autism, cancer, depression, and mental illness. Information about Vitamin D toxicity is also available on the site.

RECOMMENDED SUPPLEMENT

Bio-D-Mulsion
http://bioticsresearch.dstweb.net
Bio-D-Mulsion is a liquid vitamin D supplement that is only available from certain health care practitioners or pharmacies specializing in natural remedies. For more information, contact the manufacturer, Biotics Research Corporation, at 800-231-5777.

About the Author

Zoltan P. Rona is a graduate of McGill University Medical School and has a master's degree in biochemistry and clinical nutrition from the University of Bridgeport in Connecticut. He has had a private medical practice in Toronto for the past thirty years, is past president of the Canadian Holistic Medical Association, has appeared on radio and television, and has lectured extensively in Canada and the United States.

He is the author of three Canadian best-selling books: *The Joy of Health* (1991), *Return to the Joy of Health* (1995), and *Childhood Illness and the Allergy Connection* (1997). He is coauthor with Jeanne Marie Martin of *The Complete Candida Yeast Guidebook* (1996) and is the medical editor of the Benjamin Franklin Award-winning *Encyclopedia of Natural Healing* (1998). His latest published books in the Healthy Living Guides Series, Alive Books, include *Body Building Supplements*, *Boosting Male Libido Naturally*, *Fighting Fibromyalgia*, *Menopause Naturally*, *Natural Alternatives to Vaccination*, *Osteoarthritis Naturally*, and *Rheumatoid Arthritis Naturally*. He currently writes regular articles for *Alive*, *Revive*, and *Vitality* magazines and for several websites.

Dr. Rona is happy to answer any questions or provide more information to readers. The best way to reach him is via email at zoltan78@bellnet.ca. For more of his articles, see www.mydoctor.ca/drzoltanrona.

Index

E

F

G

H

R

S

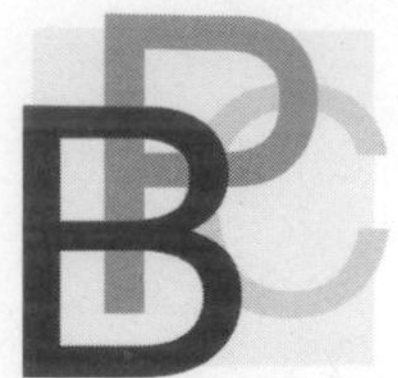

BOOK PUBLISHING COMPANY

since 1974—books that educate, inspire, and empower

To find your favorite vegetarian and soyfood products online, visit: www.healthy-eating.com

Also by Zoltan Rona, MD, MSc

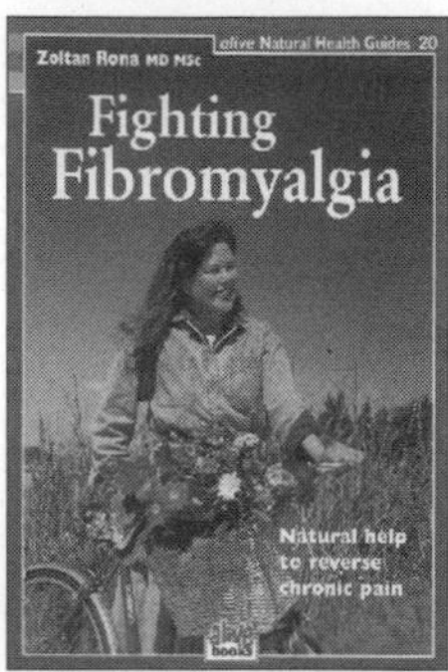

Fighting Fibromyalgia
978-1-55312-019-3
$11.95

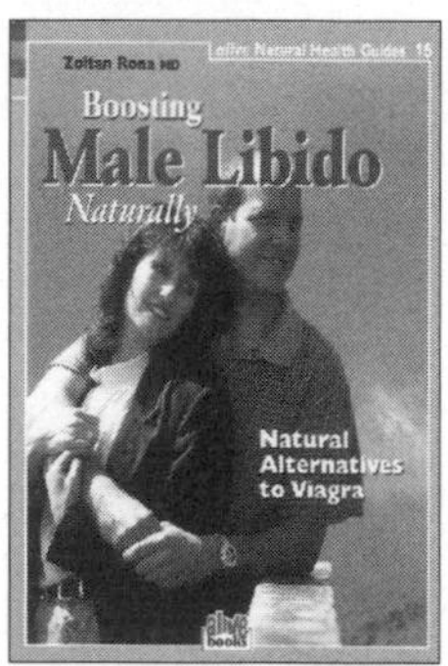

Boosting Male Libido Naturally
978-1-55312-015-5
$11.95

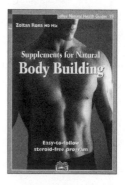

Supplements for Natural Body Building
978-1-55312-021-6
$11.95

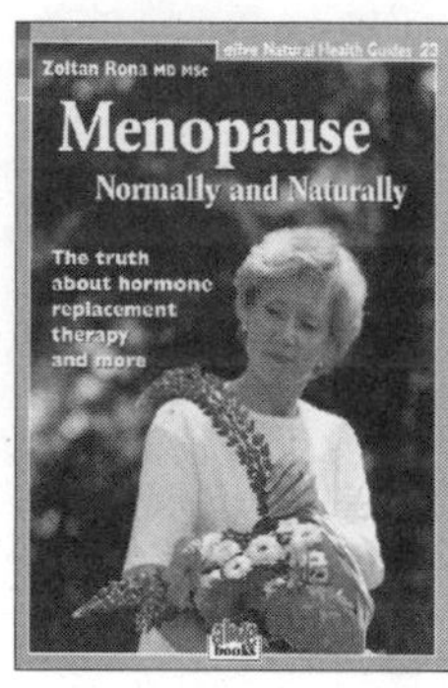

Menopause Normally and Naturally
978-1-55312-023-0
$11.95

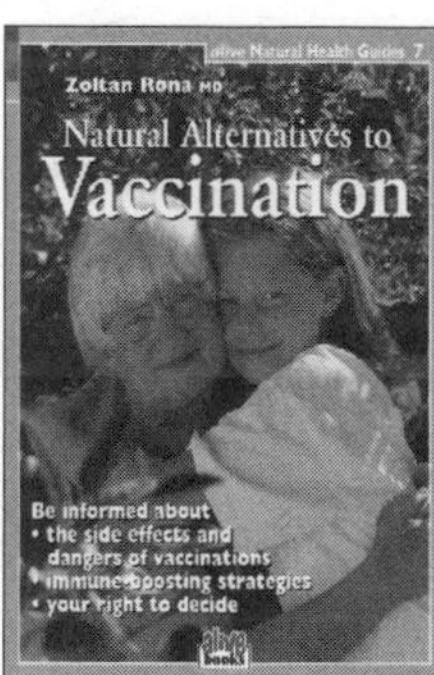

Natural Alternatives to Vaccination
978-1-55312-009-4
$11.95

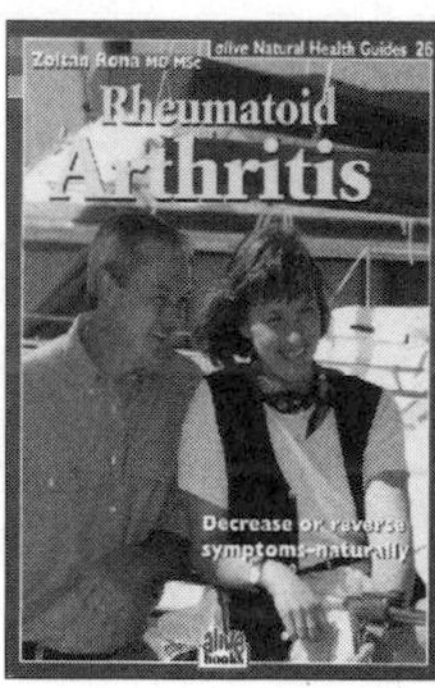

Rheumatoid Arthritis
978-1-55312-027-8
$11.95

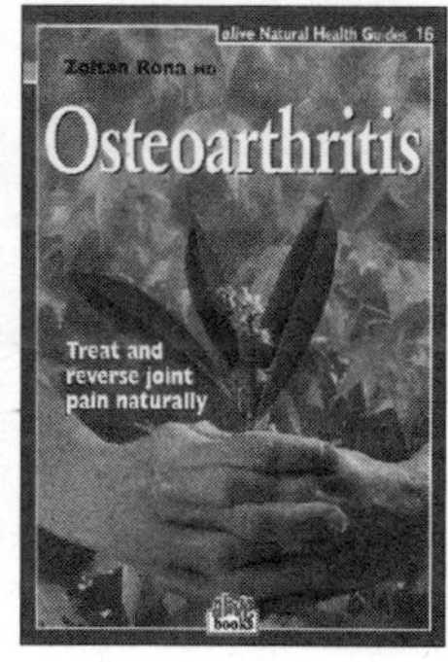

Osteoarthritis
978-1-55312-013-1
$11.95

Purchase these health titles and cookbooks from your local bookstore or natural food store, or you can buy them directly from:

Book Publishing Company • P.O. Box 99 • Summertown, TN 38483
1-800-695-2241

Please include $3.95 per book for shipping and handling.